CARING FOR A DYING LOVED ONE

Caring for a Dying Loved One

A Comprehensive Guide

BOB FISCHER, MSN, RN

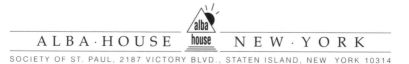

ALBA·HOUSE   NEW·YORK

SOCIETY OF ST. PAUL, 2187 VICTORY BLVD., STATEN ISLAND, NEW YORK 10314

ST PAULS

Library of Congress Cataloging-in-Publication Data

Fischer, Bob.
    Caring for a dying loved one: a comprehensive guide / Bob Fischer.
        p. cm.
    ISBN 0-8189-0896-3 (alk. paper)
        1. Terminal care—religious aspects—Catholic Church. 2. Church work with
the terminally ill—Catholic Church. 3. Caregivers—Religious life. I. Title.

    BX2347.8.S5 F57 2001
    259'.4175—dc21

                                                            2001022071

Nihil Obstat:
Rev. Isidore Dixon
Censor Deputatus

Imprimatur:
✠ Most Rev. William E. Lori, STD
Vicar General, Archdiocese of Washington, DC
May 24, 2000

Produced and designed in the United States of America by the
Fathers and Brothers of the Society of St. Paul,
2187 Victory Boulevard, Staten Island, New York 10314-6603,
as part of their communications apostolate.

ISBN: 0-8189-0896-3

Printing Information:

Current Printing - first digit	1	2	3	4	5	6	7	8	9	10

Year of Current Printing - first year shown

2001	2002	2003	2004	2005	2006	2007	2008	2009

*In loving memory of
Marian 'Tiffany', my mother,
and to all those whose hearts
she has touched in her special way.*

TABLE OF CONTENTS

ACKNOWLEDGMENTS

"Let the peace of Christ rule in your hearts, the peace to which you were called in one body. And be thankful." (Col 3:15)

I have to thank many for assistance in completing this work.

The first is the Holy Spirit, for without the grace and love of the Holy Spirit the inspiration would not have happened. It is my desire that those who read this will attain the same enlightenment that I have from the Spirit of God.

Thanks should also go to my mother, without whose love and suffering and years of loving support this book would not have been possible.

A special thanks to my good friend and Spiritual Director, Deacon Dave Cahoon, who assisted me in centering my life around the Eucharist, and whose spiritual insights helped me through many trials.

To Deacon Ron Schneider who ministers to the dying on a daily basis for his editing, cover comments, and strong support.

A special gift of love goes to the candidates and wives of the Deaconate Formation Class of 2002, Archdiocese of Washington, D.C., especially Dick, Joyce, Steve, Dodie, Perry, George, Kenneth, and Jim, for friendship and comfort during my time of grieving. A special thanks is given to Deacons Frank and Bob for their patience in putting up with such a demanding student.

I would also like to thank previous Nursing and Religious

instructors who have helped me in understanding my Christian faith.

My sister Janet played a major role in the spirituality and success in my life and helped me maintain my sanity in an otherwise insane world.

And last but certainly not least, is Karen my editor, wife, collaborator, soul mate, and best friend, who has helped me through numerous such trials.

This work of the Holy Spirit is consecrated to the Immaculate Heart of Mary for the honor and glory of her Son, Our Lord Jesus Christ and His Kingdom. "His mother said to the servers, 'Do whatever he tells you'" (Jn 2:5).

May God bless and keep all of you in the Sacred Heart of Jesus and the Immaculate Heart of Mary.

Bob

PREFACE

"What will separate us from Christ's love? Affliction,
distress, persecution, famine, destitution, danger, or the sword?
No, in all these things we are winning an overwhelming victory
through the One Who loved us." (Rm 8:35, 37)

Why did I write this easy to use guide? My mother was diagnosed with Squamos Cell lung carcinoma (cancer), which is terminal. I had experienced death many times since I was a Registered Nurse with many years of Critical Clinical Care in my background. But this was the first time I was looking into the jaws of a terminal illness with someone who was in my immediate family.

My whole world turned upside down! I was in the second year of my Deaconate Formation program in the Archdiocese of Washington D.C. when she contracted the deadly disease.

I didn't know where to start. There were many questions to which no answers were immediately available:

+ What quality of life, let alone quantity, could she expect?
+ What resources were available for her and her family?
+ What was required for the medical care of a terminally ill individual?
+ What about her last days? Was she spiritually ready?
+ What about the holy Anointing of the Sick? When could she receive that? What are Last Rites?

- According to Church teaching, did she have a right to refuse life support? Was a "Do Not Resuscitate" (DNR) order an option?
- Could life support be discontinued if already started?
- What about advanced directives and "Living Wills"? Were they acceptable?
- And what about the proper burial of a Christian?

These were difficult questions by themselves. In addition were the more personal ones of how I would be able to care for her within my hectic lifestyle. How could I take care of her on my family's income? What resources were available to me? How much was required of me in terms of Christian charity?

I was struggling between the stewardship of my own family and that of my mother with minimal resources available. What was I to do?

I recalled in the Book of Sirach, "My son, take care of your father when he is old; grieve him not as long as he lives. Even if his mind fail, be considerate with him; revile him not in the fullness of your strength."[1] I also remembered the commandment "Honor thy father and thy mother." I must help her. How?

I was torn. I had no clue what to do next and I could find no resource available for me to follow in taking care of a loved one who was dying. A lot of groundwork, research, and investigation was necessary.

I prayed "unceasingly" to the Lord for serenity, wisdom, courage, and strength. The serenity prayer that follows the preface was my direct lifeline to the Lord. I prayed that His will be done. But what was that will? What did Our Lord want me to do?

The answer came rather quickly and abruptly as I awoke from a restless sleep one morning around 3 a.m. "Write a book! Tell your story to others. Help them get through the difficulties in dealing with a dying loved one. Help others to seek My help, for 'My yoke is easy and My burden is light.'"[2]

In his letter to the Galatians, St. Paul tells us to "bear one another's burdens, and so you will fulfill the law of Christ."[3] This book is written in the hope that sharing my journey will lighten the reader's burden and make it more bearable.

Notes

[1] Si 3:12-13.
[2] Mt 11:30.
[3] Gal 6:2.

Serenity Prayer

God, grant me the serenity to accept the things I cannot change, the courage to change the things I can, and the Wisdom to know the difference.

Living one day at a time, enjoying one moment at a time. Accepting hardships as the pathway to peace. Taking as He did, this sinful world as it is, not as I would have it. Trusting that He will make all things right if I surrender to His will; that I may be reasonably happy in this life and supremely happy with Him forever. Amen.

(Alcoholics Anonymous, 12-Step Serenity Prayer)

INTRODUCTION

I Don't Know Where to Start!

"For my yoke is easy and my burden light." (Mt 11:30)

This book is a guidebook for all Christians who care for and struggle with a loved one who has become terminally ill, and for the pastoral staff who counsel them. It is intended to help the reader with the struggles of doing the Christian act of charity while balancing the responsibilities of their own life and the lives of others for whom they are responsible. This book will help the reader to address in a Christian way those issues that pop up during a terminal disease.

The book is divided into nine chapters; the format is uncomplicated and straightforward:

Chapter 1 discusses the meaning of suffering and why God permits it. It addresses the beautiful Christian view of suffering: if we offer our suffering and pain in union with Christ on the cross, then we share in His redemptive work on behalf of His Body, which is the Church. It will attempt to show how suffering, although a cross in and of itself can be a blessing.

The utilization of current theories on clinical psychological loss and grief is discussed in Chapter 2. Both the loved one who is ill and those they leave behind must go through the stages of loss and grief. Trusting in the benevolent love of God, they must come to some degree of acceptance and move forward, knowing that all things work together for the good of those who love God and submit to His Will: "For everything there is a season."[1]

The ministry of the care of the sick is addressed in Chapter 3. Section I takes up the question of whether to care for the loved one in your own home or to try to provide skilled nursing care in some other setting if necessary. This chapter will provide a thumbnail sketch of resources available and give some information needed to make this decision wisely.

Section II of Chapter 3 discusses the methods of dealing with the emotions you and other family members can expect to encounter in losing a loved one. It explains how a dying loved one can turn into an "emotional vampire," psychologically crippling the home caregiver through their manipulative behavior, and how a caregiver can best deal with them. The chapter also discusses the problem of sibling friction when families are confronted with the death of a loved one, how to prevent such friction from occurring, and the steps to take when it does occur between brothers and sisters.

Section III of Chapter 3 addresses the need to take care of the ones who care for others, and why that is so important for all involved.

The issues of resentment and anger, forgiveness and reconciliation are addressed in Chapter 4. In the Our Father we pray that God will forgive us as we forgive others. Do we really know what we are requesting when we pray this way? Do we forgive others unconditionally as we hope God forgives us? This chapter will discuss the pitfalls of resentment and the contempt it precipitates. These must be resolved before reconciliation and healing can take place.

Chapter 5 discusses the Church's teaching on bio-ethical matters as they affect decisions to be taken in caring for the sick and dying. What can and what cannot be done? When can you discontinue life support and when can you not? Is organ donation permissible? What about cremation? What about Christian burial?

"Advanced directives" such as "Do Not Resuscitate" (DNR), and "Living Wills" are also discussed. When can terminally ill individuals make decisions for themselves, and when might others have to make decisions for them?

The "last things" and preparation for the "final journey" are discussed in Chapter 6. One must prepare the soul spiritually for death. Is the person a baptized Christian? Who may receive the Lord Jesus in the Blessed Sacrament when a priest, deacon, or eucharistic minister brings Communion to the hospital room or house, and under what conditions? What about the Anointing of the Sick? Is that the same thing as the Last Rites?

Chapter 7 discusses prayer. St. Paul tells us to pray unceasingly,[2] and that the prayer of a righteous man avails much.[3] This chapter lists the types of prayer available and why it is important to pray even when one thinks that it no longer matters. Some common psalms, proverbs, and prayers to help give both the terminally ill and their caregivers comfort and solace during this difficult period are listed in Appendix B.

When your loved one is approaching imminent death, they will most likely know it. It is important for many dying individuals to be reassured that the family will be able to get along without them, and they will want to know that it is okay to die. Chapter 8 discusses why a loved one may need permission to "go home" and how a caregiver can give it. It also addresses the issues that may impede a caregiver from saying goodbye and letting go, and some methods to overcome them.

Chapter 9 brings everything together in one place. Trust in the Lord! It is in and through Him that we gain strength and comfort. Jesus tells us to "Come to me, all you who labor and are burdened, and I will give you rest. Take my yoke upon you and learn from me, for I am meek and humble of heart; and you will find rest for yourselves. For my yoke is easy, and my burden light."[4] Seek help from a friend or support person, the clergy and medical personnel. Seek help from God!

All scriptural references are from *The New Testament: St. Paul Catholic Edition* or *The New American Bible* translation unless otherwise noted.

Notes

[1] Cf. Eccl 3:1.
[2] Cf. 1 Th 5:12.
[3] Cf. Jm 5:16.
[4] Mt 11:28-30.

Biblical Abbreviations

OLD TESTAMENT

Genesis	Gn	Nehemiah	Ne	Baruch	Ba
Exodus	Ex	Tobit	Tb	Ezekiel	Ezk
Leviticus	Lv	Judith	Jdt	Daniel	Dn
Numbers	Nb	Esther	Est	Hosea	Ho
Deuteronomy	Dt	1 Maccabees	1 M	Joel	Jl
Joshua	Jos	2 Maccabees	2 M	Amos	Am
Judges	Jg	Job	Jb	Obadiah	Ob
Ruth	Rt	Psalms	Ps	Jonah	Jon
1 Samuel	1 S	Proverbs	Pr	Micah	Mi
2 Samuel	2 S	Ecclesiastes	Ec	Nahum	Na
1 Kings	1 K	Song of Songs	Sg	Habakkuk	Hab
2 Kings	2 K	Wisdom	Ws	Zephaniah	Zp
1 Chronicles	1 Ch	Sirach	Si	Haggai	Hg
2 Chronicles	2 Ch	Isaiah	Is	Malachi	Ml
Ezra	Ezr	Jeremiah	Jr	Zechariah	Zc
		Lamentations	Lm		

NEW TESTAMENT

Matthew	Mt	Ephesians	Eph	Hebrews	Heb
Mark	Mk	Philippians	Ph	James	Jm
Luke	Lk	Colossians	Col	1 Peter	1 P
John	Jn	1 Thessalonians	1 Th	2 Peter	2 P
Acts	Ac	2 Thessalonians	2 Th	1 John	1 Jn
Romans	Rm	1 Timothy	1 Tm	2 John	2 Jn
1 Corinthians	1 Cor	2 Timothy	2 Tm	3 John	3 Jn
2 Corinthians	2 Cor	Titus	Tt	Jude	Jude
Galatians	Gal	Philemon	Phm	Revelation	Rv

CARING FOR A DYING LOVED ONE

1

WHY DOES GOD PERMIT SUFFERING?
The Meaning of Suffering

"The Spirit itself bears witness with our spirit that we are God's children. And if we are children, then we are also heirs, heirs of God and co-heirs with Christ, if we suffer with him so as to be glorified with him as well." (Rm 8:17)

Does God enjoy watching us suffer? Why doesn't He stop all the evil in the world? How can a loving compassionate God permit these things to happen?

God does not enjoy suffering and evil; in fact, He abhors it. He is not detached from it since His only begotten Son suffered and died on the cross for our sins. He knows suffering firsthand. He suffered because He loves us unconditionally. So why does He allow evil and suffering if He loves us so much?

It is *because* He loves us that He allows evil and suffering. God in His plan for eternity created us with *free will*. When Adam and Eve, our first parents, abused their free will and pridefully sinned against God, all of their descendants developed an inherent propensity to sin. Evil begets evil, and the more evil there is in the world, the more need there is to turn back to God in prayer and repentance to make reparation for sin.

Physical evil such as disease and natural disasters also entered the world as a result of Original Sin. Why, we ask ourselves, do so many people die and suffer as a result of these events? Does God like to see us suffer? No, these events occur as natural phenomena. God does not allow these events in order that we might suffer and die from them. In fact, "on the cross Christ took upon himself the whole weight of evil… of which illness is only a consequence. By his passion and death on the cross, Christ has given a new meaning to suffering: it can henceforth configure us to him and unite us with his redemptive Passion" (*Catechism*, 1505). Another positive side to major disasters in the world is that people of good will are drawn together to help one another in the spirit of Christian charity, and in the process, many people turn to God. God oftentimes takes evil events and brings good out of them.

Some say that God should warn us when a disaster is imminent. How do we know that He doesn't try to warn us? How many times do we get an uneasy feeling about something only to ignore it and do the opposite? The result can be disastrous. Many times we hear stories of people who for whatever reason miss their plane, only to have it go down in a ball of flames sometime later. When asked how they made the decision to turn back, they could only reply that "something told me not to get onboard." In many ways Jesus talks to our hearts on a daily basis, but we choose not to listen or we ignore Him because it is not what we want to do or hear. We harden our hearts so that we are unable to listen to Jesus. "Oh, that today you would hear his voice: 'Harden not your hearts.'"[1]

But why can't God just prevent bad things from happening all together? Think about this scenario for a moment: Living in a world without pain and suffering, where everything is just wonderful. Nothing to worry about or to fret over. How long would we need God in our lives? Why should we seek heaven when we have heaven on earth? To make things worse, we would not even give God the credit for it all. It would have been just a lucky break for us. We blame God for the suffering and evil in the world, but we never give Him credit or thank Him for the happiness and good.

THE MEANING OF SUFFERING

But what of my aunt who is dying of lung disease? What evil has she done? Why is God allowing her to suffer?

The question for Christians here is not why God is allowing suffering, but what kind of meaning can be derived from suffering.

A universal meaning for suffering is almost impossible to define. There are many different kinds of suffering and each person suffers in an individual way. There is, however, one maxim that generally applies to all of us: We need suffering to develop as adults. We don't know what we can bear if we don't experience it. Without pain and suffering in our lives, we cannot adequately appreciate happiness and joy.

What possible good can come from suffering? What possible rational meaning can we derive from it? Viktor Frankl, a Holocaust survivor, psychotherapist, and author of *Meaning of Human Suffering* said, "Suffering ceases to be when one finds a meaning for it."[2]

THE CHRISTIAN MEANING OF SUFFERING

As Christians, we are called to share in the suffering of Christ. "Jesus said to his disciples, 'Whoever would be my disciple must deny himself, take up his cross, and follow me.'"[3] St. Paul tells us, "God has graciously allowed you not only to believe in Christ but also to suffer for him."[4] Again, Christ tells us that if we suffer with Him and in His name, we will also be glorified with

Him.[5] If we suffer in accordance with God's will, we will entrust our souls to a faithful Creator and do good.[6]

The Christian view of suffering brings with it the most beautiful consolation that a person who suffers can enjoy. We, who suffer in the name of Christ as members of His mystical body, share in His redemptive work. "I rejoice in what I am suffering for your sake now, and in my flesh I am completing what is lacking in Christ's afflictions on behalf of his body, that is, the church."[7]

In his Apostolic Letter on Salvific Suffering, *Salvifici Doloris,* Pope John Paul II says, "The Redeemer suffered in place of man and for man. Every man has his own share in the Redemption. Each one is also called to share in that suffering through which the Redemption was accomplished. He is called to share in that suffering through which all human suffering has also been redeemed. In bringing about the Redemption through suffering, Christ has also raised human suffering to the level of the Redemption. Thus each man, in his suffering, can also become a sharer in the Redemptive suffering of Christ."[8]

GIVE MEANING TO YOUR SUFFERING

The meaning of suffering is not to be found in the "Why me, why now?" questions. It can, however, be found in the questions, "What can I do with my suffering?" and "How can I benefit from the situation given to me?" This is best answered by the Christian belief that in doing God's will we are ultimately blessed.[9] Offer up your suffering and the suffering of those you love for the eternal salvation of others.

We can offer our suffering for those who need our prayers. In this selfless act of Christian charity, we enter into the suffering and death of Jesus and a share in His eternal life and glory!

Can you find a more beautiful meaning for suffering than God allowing us the privilege to intercede for the eternal good of others?

Jesus allows those He loves to suffer in and with Him. On Calvary, Jesus allowed His mother to bear the weight of His suffering beneath the cross. As Simeon had foretold, "(and a sword will pierce your own soul), so that the thoughts of many hearts may be revealed."[10]

We have the perfect model of how to suffer in Jesus. "This is what you were called to, and this is why Christ suffered for you, to leave you an example for you to follow in his footsteps."[11]

A MYSTERY PARTIALLY RESOLVED

We may never fully understand why a loving God would allow suffering and pain. It will be a mystery to us until the time when we behold the glory of Jesus face to face. One thing certain is that mysteries are for Jesus to reveal. We as humans cannot solve them alone. But Jesus helps us to understand the mystery by giving meaning to our suffering: the honor to share in His redemptive work.

Ask the Holy Spirit to give you and your suffering loved ones the graces needed to endure. Offer your suffering in reparation for your sins and those of others who are unable or unwilling to do so.

Notes

[1] Heb 4:7.
[2] Viktor E. Frankl, *Meaning of Human Suffering* (Boston: Beacon Press, 1985).
[3] Mt 16:24.
[4] Ph 1:29.

5 Cf. Rm 8:17.

6 1 P 4:19.

7 Col 1:24.

8 John Paul II, Apostolic Letter *Salvifici Doloris* (February 11, 1984), 19.

9 Leo E. Missinne, *How To Find Meaning in Suffering* (Liguori, MO: Liguori Press, 1990), pp. 18-19.

10 Lk 2:35.

11 1 P 2:21.

2

BLESSED ARE THEY WHO MOURN

Stages of Grief and Loss

*"There is an appointed time for everything,
and a time for every affair under the heavens. A time to be born,
and a time to die; a time to plant, and a time to
uproot the plant."* (Ec 3:1-2)

In the previous chapter, the meaning of suffering and an acceptable, if not fully adequate, answer to why God permits suffering was briefly discussed. Illness can result in a type of suffering that goes beyond the loss of one's health to include many other kinds of loss: loss of control, familiarity, friendships, relationships, family, mobility, happiness, and even one's life when the illness is terminal.

All human beings suffer some form of loss. A middle-aged man suffers the loss of his job to a younger man. The poor suffer the lack of money, adequate housing, food, clothing and medical care. Families mourn the death of a pet. No suffering, however, comes close to equaling that of the loss of a human life. A man dies from the complications of Acquired Immune Deficiency Syndrome (AIDS), but he is not alone in his suffering. His wife suffers the loss of her husband and his child mourns the loss of her father. Whole families suffer when a loved one is terminally ill. The country mourns the death of its servicemen and women who give their lives in the course of duty.

Grieving is the natural process by which we are healed after such a loss. We all grieve differently and for different reasons, but we all go through with the same basic steps, symptoms, feelings, and emotions. Diagram #1 illustrates this process.

THE GRIEVING PROCESS

As the diagram illustrates, grieving is a *dynamic* process which in general goes through three stages. The boxes represent the different stages of grief due to loss or imminent loss as a result of terminal illness: (1) *Denial and Anger*, (2) *Bargaining and Disorganization*, and (3) *Reorganization*. The bi-directional arrows between the boxes indicate the pathways followed in the process. The arrow direction suggests that as we go forward in healing, a situation, person, or thing can cause us to regress to an earlier stage of healing.

The areas inside the boxes indicate feelings and emotions that are common at each stage. The dialogue boxes indicate the physical, mental and social symptoms associated with these feelings and emotions. Feelings, emotions, and symptoms are oftentimes present from the previous or next stages, indicating that there is an undifferentiated progression from one stage to the other.

LOSS

DENIAL /ANGER

Feelings / Emotions
Relief, fear, denial, anger, shock, guilt, rejection, decreased self-esteem

Symptoms
Overly sensitive, numbness, crying, aches, weakness, pain, sleep disturbance, appetite disturbance, overly dependent, irritable.

Symptoms
Susceptibility to illness, restlessness, decreased socialization, physical symptoms, delayed thinking and reactions, confusion, forgetfulness, need to recover what was lost.

BARGAINING /DISORGANIZATION

Feelings / Emotions
Sadness, loneliness, withdrawal, inhibitions, apathy, anxiety, bargaining, anguish, depression.

REORGANIZATION

Feelings / Emotions
Pleasure, increased energy, increased self-esteem, reaching out to others.

Symptoms
Return to level of function, increased social activity, improved self-image, gradual loss of persistent memories of the loved one.

Acceptance and Moving On!

THE FEELINGS AND EMOTIONS OF GRIEF

Every human grieves a loss of one form or another. Even Jesus grieved at the death of Lazarus and mourned for John the Baptist.[1] The loss or imminent loss of a loved one or thing creates an emptiness, void, or vacuum inside of us. It takes away something that once was and is no longer. It takes away our ability to control our lives. We are left vulnerable to others and all that the misfortunes of life can bring.

As we grieve our loss and start the long process towards healing, we can expect to feel all the emotions in each of the following steps, and to manifest all the symptoms. As stated above, grieving is a dynamic process with progress often being followed by regression and vice versa. All it takes is for a scent, a picture, a holiday, an anniversary, a memory of the loss to put the wheels of progress in reverse. This is a normal part of the healing process. It helps us to cope with those realities that we believe we will never be able to handle.

Denial/Anger

When the loss of our own lives or that of a loved one threatens, we cannot bring ourselves to believe that this could ever happen to us. Things like this happen to other people. We deny the fact and often become angry. The feelings we experience are fear, denial, anger, shock, guilt, confusion, rejection, and decreased self-esteem. As we work through this process we become overly sensitive and irritable. We manifest many or all of the symptoms of numbness, crying, aches and pains, weakness, and sleep disturbances.

Bargaining/Disorganization

In this stage, we start making "deals" with God and others. "If you take this disease away I will go to church more often." "I will say more Rosaries." "I'll be a better person if you let me or my loved one live." "Why can't you give this trial to my co-worker instead; she can handle it better than I?" "Can I lick this disease if I eat better and exercise?"

Our lives become more chaotic and disorganized as we are forced to deal with the reality of what lies ahead. The feelings we experience are sadness, loneliness, withdrawal, apathy, anxiety, bargaining, anguish, inhibitions and depression. During this time we find ourselves susceptible to illness, increased restlessness, decreased socialization, physical symptoms such as delayed thinking and reactions, confusion, forgetfulness, and the need to recover what was lost.

Reorganization

It is during this stage following the loss of a loved one that life regains a semblance of normality. The loss is no longer as devastating as it once was and you realize that although the pain does not entirely go away, you can deal with it. You are on the road to recovery. Feelings and emotions during this stage are those of increased energy, self-esteem, pleasure, and a desire to reach out to others. There is a return to a more normal level of functioning, increased social activities, the gradual loss of persistent memories of the loved one, improved self-image, and a movement toward total healing.

What Can I Do to Heal?

The first thing to do is to trust in God, even if it seems impossible or illogical to do so at this time. All our strength comes from God. Prayer is essential. Pray as often as you can and wherever you can. The following course of action can aid you in the healing process.

♦ *Let Yourself Experience the Grieving Process* — The ability to love includes the capacity to grieve the loss of those we love. Yes, grieving hurts, but you cannot heal properly if you do not grieve. Healing is a process and it takes time. Take one day at a time, enjoy one moment at a time as you are able. Say the *Serenity Prayer* whenever you feel the need of encouragement, strength, courage, or wisdom.

♦ *Grieve In Your Own Way* — No one grieves like you do. No two people grieve in the same way. Each person has his or her own unique sense of loss, unique set of personal circumstances, unique support system, and unique religious and cultural background. What might be extremely painful for one person is just an annoyance to another. Do not let anyone tell you how you should grieve.

♦ *Talk About Your Grief* — Verbalizing your grief prevents you from keeping it boxed up inside where it can do you harm. Talking about it won't get rid of the grief, but it will make you feel better. Seek a caring friend, relative or support person who is willing to listen and not just "hear."

♦ *Lean On Your Support System* — In times of grief it is important to have a good support system. It can be difficult to reach out to others especially when you feel so disorganized. You need to do so, however. Seek friends and family members with whom you can easily talk in both happy times and sad. It is helpful to find someone who has been through a similar loss to walk through the grieving process with you. You may also wish to seek out a pastor, priest, or deacon.

♦ *Find Meaning in Your Suffering* — Viktor Frankl, a survivor of the Holocaust, found that "Suffering ceases to be when one finds a meaning for it."[2] Find a trusted friend to discuss your thoughts with. Remember, as Christians we share in Christ's redemptive work in His Church by offering our sufferings in union with His and for the sake of others.

♦ *Try to Maintain Your Health and Sense of Humor* — This is logically the most important point. You cannot help others if you are sick yourself. The care of the dying individual can be very draining, both emotionally and physically. Take time to care for yourself, the caregiver.

HEALING IS A PROCESS

Grief is a natural response to the loss of someone that we love or cherish. It is an indicator that this person truly held a special place in our hearts. Just as we are all different in how we grieve, we are also different in the length of time in which we grieve. It may take a few months to as many as two years or more to work through the process. Some people go straight through the stages while others periodically regress to earlier stages and have to repeat some of the steps. We must work through all of the stages of grieving if we are to heal.

Treasure the memories you have of your family member or friend. Dr. Wolfelt, author of the article, "Twelve Freedoms of Healing in Grief," tells us that we have the "right or freedom" to treasure our memories. "Memories are one of the best legacies that exist after someone loved dies."[3] Memories are the lasting part of the relationship that we had with our loved one who has passed on.

Have faith in the Lord. Remember what Jesus said, "Come to me, all you grown weary and burdened, and I will refresh you. Take my yoke upon you and learn from me, for I am gentle and humble of heart; and you will find rest for your souls. For my yoke is easy, and my burden light."[4] Fill yourself with the hope and joy of the risen Christ. Mother Teresa of Calcutta once said, "Never let anything so fill you with sorrow as to make you forget the joy of Christ risen."

Notes

[1]   Cf. Jn 11:32-36; Mt 14:13.
[2]   Frankl, *Meaning of Human Suffering.*
[3]   Alan D. Wolfelt, "Twelve Freedoms of Healing in Grief," *Bereavement Magazine* (February 1993), pp. 35-36.
[4]   Mt 11:28-30.

3

A CHARITABLE MINISTRY

Caring for the Sick and Dying

"I am able to do everything through the One Who strengthens me."
(Ph 4:13)

The diagnosis of a terminal disease affects not only the person with the illness but also all those whose hearts have been touched by that person in their life. It particularly affects the immediate family. When the person who is ill is dying, a piece of each member of the family dies along with them.

Coping with the terminal illness of someone you love is an all-consuming affair. It takes much energy and drains physical, emotional, mental, and financial resources in the process. How do you deal with all the special needs, emotions, and wishes of the dying family member or friend? How do you give them the permission to "go on" when you would rather they stay behind? It is distressing to watch someone you love die. A part of you wants to die with them. You may even bargain that it be you instead.

You must be prepared. Many times family and friends will depend on you to make decisions on their behalf. They will ask you many questions. Where do you go for answers? What resources are available to help? And how do you care for the caregivers?

This chapter will address these questions in three sections. Section I will discuss how to choose a place to provide care for the terminally ill patient. The challenges of dealing with emotions and feelings of the dying are discussed in Section II. In Section III, the care of the home caregiver and the family is discussed. While caring for the dying can be physically and emotionally draining, it can also be very fulfilling and rewarding.

I. MAKING A DECISION ON PROVIDING CARE

How and where do you care for someone who can no longer care for him or herself? Will the person need a skilled nursing facility, hospice or respite center, or can the family take care of them at home? The answer depends on the patient's condition, wishes, the environment, emotional and financial resources, and the capability and readiness of the family.

Two Scenarios

Jane has just spent two stressful weeks at the hospital bedside of her mom undergoing treatment for cancer. The social worker planning her discharge now says that mom has to leave because she has no further need for the type of care given in a hospital. The social worker wants to know where mom will be discharged. Where does mom go from here?

Scenario 1

Jane would like to take mom into her home and care for her. But mom needs to be watched 24 hours a day. Neither Jane nor her husband can afford to leave work because they are dependent on both incomes.

Under normal circumstances, Jane could probably take leave time to care for mom, but she used the last of her leave to be at mom's bedside during her treatments. Jane's two teenage daughters are away at college and Jane has tuition fees to pay. Jane is an only child and there is no one else who could help in mom's care.

Jane makes the decision that mom must go into a nursing home. Jane knew of one near her home that had a good reputation, and she could spend much more time at her mother's side if she were to go there.

Scenario 2

Jane, a mother of two teenage girls, is financially secure. Jane has a small savings account that she had started for just such an emergency. With her two teenage daughters, and a little custodial care from hospice, Jane can comfortably take mom into her home and provide for 24-hour care.

Jane has discussed it with her husband and her daughters and a plan of action has been drawn up with the help of the physician, hospice nursing staff, and social workers. Everyone has been assigned a duty and responsibility and is prepared to care for Jane's mom at home.

Which Scenario is Preferable?

They both are. In each scenario, Jane is doing the best she can under the circumstances. There is no absolute answer to this question and there are additional scenarios that could yet be considered.

If you are responsible for the care of a family member or friend with a terminal illness, you may have to make these decisions. The next few sections will assist you in doing so.

Care in a Skilled Nursing Facility

Some of your family, friends, and co-workers may question why you do not chose home care. Although it is generally preferable for most people to die in the familiar surroundings of home and family, this simply may not be possible. Decisions must be made and there are no absolute answers. Don't let anyone coerce you into making a decision which you are not emotionally, physically, or financially capable of making.

There is some important information that you need to know, however, before you place your loved one in a skilled nursing care facility. Some facilities may be filled to capacity and there may be a waiting list for admission. This is especially true for those facilities that are popular or have an established reputation. Other facilities are sub-standard and you may not feel comfortable placing your loved one in such a place.

Many private health insurance plans won't cover admission to skilled nursing facilities unless there is a special "rider" to the insurance policy. Medicare may only cover admission for a set number of days, depending on the illness. Private health insurance and/or Medicaid may pick up the remainder, but Medicaid has specific criteria. Social workers are trained to deal with these issues. Please be thorough in checking your case out with a social worker or patient advocate.

Care at Home

If it is within your ability to do so, there is nothing more beautiful than taking care of a loved one who is terminally ill in the familiar sights, smells, and surroundings of home. Many people consider this a more natural way of dying than in the sterility and unfamiliar surroundings of a health care institution.

A few things, nonetheless, need to be considered. Your

loved one may require round-the-clock care. They may require special medications, oxygen, medical equipment, medical supplies, and the like. Round-the-clock means care during all hours of the day and night. Dying people sometimes get their times confused, staying awake during the night and sleeping during the day. This can be quite fatiguing to the caregivers, who generally must still lead an active life as well.

The room that the loved ones occupy may not be amenable to the care they need or may be too small. Many dying loved ones have had to spend their remaining days on a hospital bed in the middle of a family or living room.

Even given all the above considerations, most people who have taken care of the dying at home relate how it is the best and most rewarding thing they ever have done, and that they would do it again if they had to. There are resources to help those caring for a loved one at home, many of which are listed in Appendix A of this book. One of the most valuable resources for terminally ill patients is the *hospice program*.

The Hospice Team: A Valuable Resource

What is *hospice*? Hospice is a program run by a team of professionals who are prepared to deal with the special needs of dying patients and their families. The team may vary from state to state or county to county. In general, the team consists of a physician (oftentimes an oncologist or other specialist), registered nurses, home health aides, social workers, chaplains, and volunteers. The patient's personal physician frequently remains as a consultant. The team stays involved with the patient and family during the final days of the illness and continues to provide the family bereavement support for up to a year after the death of the patient.

Hospice programs provide a plan of care that has been decided on by the patient, family, personal physician, and the hospice team. Generally the following is provided by all hospice programs in the home or in approved hospice centers:

- Regularly scheduled visits by a Registered Nurse
- A 24-hour on-call RN
- Home health aides to assist with personal care
- Social services and counseling
- Volunteer support for patient and caregivers
- Illness awareness and education
- Medical equipment, supplies, and medication which are related to the terminal illness
- Short term round-the-clock medical care
- Pastoral Care Services
- Bereavement support

Enrollment is covered 100% by Medicare and Medicaid nationwide, and most private health insurance plans likewise cover it. The criteria for acceptance generally are met if the patient is determined by their personal physician to have a terminal disease with a prognosis of six months or less to live, and all means of curative therapy have been exhausted or become futile. This does not mean that after six months the patient is booted out of the program. If the personal physician and the hospice team document terminal disease progression, it can and usually does get covered longer for the extent of the disease progression or death.

Is Hospice the Right Choice for Your Needs?

Hospice may not be appropriate for all situations. Is your situation such that you should ask the hospice team into your home? Here are a few criteria to help you decide.

♦ Has the physician exhausted every treatment that will cure the illness or prolong a dignified and meaningful life?

♦ Has the loved one been given a terminal prognosis of six months or less?

♦ Is the loved one aware of his terminal illness? What about the rest of the family? The hospice team should not surprise the patient with a diagnosis that he or she is not prepared to accept.

♦ Are family and friends willing to assist in the 24/7 care a terminal patient will need?

♦ Does the patient desire to remain in the familiar surroundings of home while he/she is dying?

Hospice care is an indispensable resource if you are planning to take care of your loved one at home. There is no reason to tough it out on your own. Your physician, staff nurse, or social worker will give you information about hospice programs in your area. You can call or write one of the hospice resources listed in Appendix A.

II. Dealing with the Feelings of the Dying Person

This section will guide you in handling the ever-changing emotions of a dying person. Many times emotional outbursts from a dying loved one cause resentment, anger, and hurt feelings. But it need not be this way if one understands the pathology behind the feelings and emotions these individuals are exhibiting. Taking each stage of loss and grief mentioned in the previous chapter, here are some guidelines in better dealing with them.

Denial/Anger

"Denial is the refusal to accept reality, and grows out of shock."[1] It can be manifested in many ways. For instance, "I don't believe you. I want a second opinion," or, "Impossible, there is no cancer in my family," or, "Not me! I'm going to beat this."

The best way to handle denial is to compassionately address the denial. Don't force the person to accept their fate, but at the same time, don't encourage their illusion. Recognize the underlying desire behind the denial. If an individual tells you that they will get better and that we can go skiing again, respond by saying "Wouldn't we have fun?"[2] Don't take away their hope, but don't feed their illusion.

A dying individual may feel anger for many reasons. Although most times not intentional, anger can be directed towards loved ones. What makes a dying person angry? The most common things are loss of control, resentment, and fear.

Loss of Control

Loss of control and the frustration it causes is a major factor. A dying person loses control over his life. This makes him or her frustrated and angry, and that anger may be directed towards you.

Try to recognize the underlying helplessness in their life and make an effort to address it. Give your loved one as much control in their lives as possible. Let them choose, if possible, the times they will be washed, eat, etc. You cannot give them back their life, but you can give them back some control of it.

Resentment

Loss of control leads to *resentment*. "Why am I dying and you are still alive to enjoy the things I used to? I resent that! That makes me so angry!" Try to avoid or defuse situations or actions that would be resented by the dying loved one. For instance, if grandma enjoyed knitting sweaters so much that she showed you how to do it, don't knit sweaters in front of her if you feel that it bothers her.

The patient may also resent his or her own body. There may have been a time when the condition or shape of their body had meant everything to them. Now what they once may have cherished is betraying them.

Fear

Some people won't or can't put their fears into words, and consequently act them out. They might have fear about pain, fear of dying alone, and fear of the unknown. Even a person who is a Christian when facing death may have doubts about the "real" existence of God.

Try to identify what these fears are by just listening. Dispel any rumors, and offer the help of a pastor, priest, or deacon to discuss any issues of faith. Most fears can be overcome if people face them, but don't force them to face their fears if they don't want to or are not ready to.

Bargaining

Bargaining is an attempt by the dying person to postpone the inevitable. They try to bargain with God to get rid of this nasty illness. "If you take this away from me, I will donate more time to helping the poor." Many will say, "If I eat well and stick to my treatments, the cancer will go away." People who have contracted AIDS may make deals to spend the time they have left working to stop AIDS from spreading.[3]

If bargaining does occur, it is usually not known by others.

If it is told to you, just treat it with respect and suggest that it would be great if that will happen. To do anything else would be to shoot down any hope the loved one has.

Disorganization

Clinical depression can follow from grief. The terminally ill are mourning what they have already lost by their illness and what will be lost when they die.[4]

The loved one's life has been turned upside down. They become disjointed, disorganized. Do not take this lightly and do not downplay it. The best thing you can do is listen and let them ventilate their thoughts.

Reorganization/Acceptance

Acceptance is a peaceful resignation by the loved one to the inevitable. It usually comes to them closer to death. Their lives become more organized and things seem brighter and clearer.

Occasionally, an event, holiday, or memory will cause the person to regress to another stage as death approaches. The best thing to do is to provide love and comfort at this point. It is important to note that when a loved one has peace and acceptance, it may come with detachment from others. This can be hard for the loved ones left behind to accept.[5]

The "Emotional Vampire"

We all know at least one of these. These are the people who let you know, no matter what you do, it is not good enough. They are not content until they "suck" the last bit of energy from you. Nothing you do is right and everything you do is wrong. They know how to "push your buttons" or "pull your strings," and they do it very well. They are experts at it! The "emotional vampire" can convert the home caregiver into an "emotional cripple."

The emotional vampires can be the emotionally dysfunctional, mentally unstable, or demented loved ones. They are difficult to deal with in the best of times, but can be little less than a nightmare when they are sick. They are generally self-centered, co-dependent, demanding, materialistic, paranoid, angry, controlling, hateful… the list goes on and on. In their self-centeredness, for whatever the pathology, they believe the world exists for and through them alone. When they cannot live life on their own terms they become very frustrated and act out their frustration.

Dealing with the "Emotional Vampire"

The first thing that you must keep reminding yourself — no matter how angry or frustrated you get — is that this person is dying and needs your unconditional love. Remember that Jesus loved us unconditionally even as we were crucifying Him on the cross: "Father forgive them, they know not what they do!"[6]

You treat the symptoms of grief as above, but you must set limits. Limits include the limits you set on others and on yourself. Cloud and Townsend equate limits with boundaries. They state that boundary setting involves making your own choices and taking responsibility for them.[7]

When setting limits you let the loved one know that a certain behavior upsets you, that you will not tolerate that behavior and what will happen if the behavior continues to the limit set. You then do what you said you would if the behavior continues.

Example:

Mother, you know when you (*insert behavior here*) that it really upsets me. All I want to do right now is give you all the love I have, but I cannot give you my all if you continue to upset me by (*insert behavior here*). Therefore, if you continue to (*insert behavior here*) I will (*insert consequence of behavior*).

It is important to note that you must be prepared to carry out the consequence of the behavior as stated. To fail to do so will show the loved one that you are not serious and that will just give them another "button to push" or "string to pull."

Anger and Guilt

Setting limits takes some control away from the loved one, and as mentioned above, loss of control leads to anger. The loved one will act out this anger and try to regain control any way they can. This acting out may and most times does include guilt messages, such as "How can you abandon me like this?" or "You never loved me anyway."

They may even try to attack your spirituality such as, "A 'real' Christian wouldn't do this to their mother" or "Doesn't the Bible say honor you parents?" They will resist this limit setting at all costs. How can you deal with resistance to limit setting and still allow the loved one to maintain the degree of control needed for the grieving process?

Dealing with Resistance to Limit Setting

Anger and guilt messages are common obstacles to limit setting. Cloud and Townsend give the following advice for dealing with resistance to setting boundaries.[8]

Angry Reactions

The angry person has a personality problem. If reinforced, it will come back again and again. They feel as though they are "owed" things from others and when they don't get them, they lose a part of their control. What should you do?

♦ Realize that the one who has the problem is the person who is angry with you.
♦ Anger cannot hurt you unless you let it. *[ß u!]*
♦ Do not let anger decide your course for you. Let the person be angry and you be the navigator of the course of action.
♦ Use your support systems to help you decide on a course of action.
♦ Love the person who is angry with you and don't allow them to evoke your anger.
♦ Allow yourself space when you feel threatened.
♦ Empathize, not sympathize, with the angry person and try to defuse their anger without being controlled by it.
♦ Learn what 'things' push your buttons or pull your strings and try to defuse them ahead of time.
♦ Remember that God loves unconditionally and so should you. When Jesus was gasping for His last breath on the cross He begged the Father to "forgive them, for they do not know what they do."[9] He still loved those around Him, even while they mocked, ridiculed and crucified Him.

Guilt Messages

Your loved one tells you, "You don't love me anymore, do you?" You are going out of your way to show love for this person, but they do not seem to recognize it. Cloud and Townsend offer the following tips.[10]

♦ Recognize that messages directed at you are guilt messages.
♦ Anger is the underlying purpose of a guilt message.
♦ People send guilt messages because they are sad and they hurt.

- ◆ If your buttons are pushed by a guilt message, it becomes your problem, not your loved one's.
- ◆ You do not have to justify your actions.
- ◆ Recognize guilt messages as being about feelings and not a personal affront to you.

Limit setting is important when the loved one is manipulative. Be assured that the loved one will probably not allow you to take away the control they have on you. It will be difficult, but you must set limits for both you and your loved one if you are to maintain your sanity through it all.

Sibling Friction

Another matter to consider is sibling rivalry or more appropriately, "sibling friction." Children of a sick parent, even those who are very close and loving to one another, sometimes develop conflicts, tensions, arguments and even fist fights over who can do the "best job" in caring for the parent. This is especially true of the parent who lives alone.

Otherwise loving brothers and sisters can develop jealousies when mom moves in with the other sibling to spend her last days, or when one sibling likes a specific nursing facility more than the one chosen by the other. The issue of geographic distance can compound this problem.

Arguments can arise over the need for extraordinary treatment (discussed in Chapter 5) or the desired burial arrangements of the children if the parent has not specified his or her desires. Add to this a child who may be experiencing guilt due to the fact that he or she may not have been a "loving" child through the years.

It is unfortunate but the death of a parent, like any other major stress on the family, can bring out the worst in children. There may even be a resurfacing of long resolved childhood conflicts. What can be done to prevent or at least minimize this problem?

Resolving Sibling Friction

It is inevitable that some degree of sibling friction will occur. This friction must be defused and resolved as soon as possible to prevent additional stress, hurt, and resentment. You should start by making a plan.

- ♦ Try to identify those areas where there might be potential issues or conflicts with siblings in the care of the parent.
- ♦ Identify an impartial third party to intervene when problems arise. Together a family chooses a third party who can "see the forest in spite of the trees" and intervene when friction starts to occur. When my sister and I started to attack each other, my father, long divorced from my mother, stepped in. He analyzed the situation and defused it before it even got a chance to take hold by identifying the issues involved and helping us to resolve them. This may or may not have been possible without an "arbitrator" of some sort and the issues may have been blown out of control and jeopardized the loving relationship that I enjoyed with my sister.
- ♦ Discuss and make major decisions involving the care of the parent together when possible. This may not always be practical in that some decisions need to be made immediately without time for consulting the other siblings. In the latter situation, keep the others informed of all major decisions and milestones as they occur. But whenever possible, decide together on the best possible course of action.
- ♦ Forgive all childhood conflicts, tensions, and resentments and reconcile if possible. Learn to forgive and be forgiven as discussed in Chapter 4.

♦ Pray unceasingly. God will help you if you ask Him. Pray for serenity, courage, and wisdom that as a family you may endure the hardships ahead, and grow more spiritually in Him.

III. CARING FOR THE HOME CAREGIVER

Whatever method of care you decide on, your family needs to pull together and support each other.

♦ Learn all you can about the illness so that you are better prepared to accept whatever comes your way. (Lists of organizations are in Appendix A.)

♦ Recognize the signs and symptoms of grief and loss. Be tolerant of the patient's requests, desires, and needs but set limits. A dying person deserves your attention but over coddling can be more hurtful than helpful. Learn to set attainable limits.

♦ Talk to each other. Share your concerns, disappointments, joys, and setbacks. Be open and frank but be gentle and kind. Remember that the other members of your family are suffering also.

♦ Prepare a "plan of action." Assign each person a duty and responsibility. But also make sure that each caregiver is cared for. It does the sick loved one no good if the caregivers become ill. Provide and take every opportunity for rest and relaxation, watch your diet, and make sure you exercise.

♦ Maintain your lifestyle as normally as possible. Your job is to be there for the loved one, not to overpower and overprotect them. If your family members enjoy going to dance rehearsals, or bowling with the boys, or belonging to Church functions, try to maintain that lifestyle as best as possible.

It is part of your relaxation and socialization/support process. You owe it to yourself and the ones you love.

♦ Let your faith in God help you. God is there to give you strength. Maintain your ties with Church groups, especially prayer and Bible study groups. Ask for prayers from other people. Go to Mass and receive the sacraments more frequently. And fit time into your life for prayer.

♦ When it is time to say goodbye, let go. This will be discussed in Chapter 8.

Notes

1. Maggie Callanan and Patricia Kelley, *Final Gifts* (NY: Bantam Books, 1997), p. 39.
2. *Ibid.*, p. 40.
3. *Ibid.*, p. 50.
4. *Ibid.*
5. *Ibid.*, p. 52.
6. Lk 23:34.
7. Henry Cloud and John Townsend, *Boundaries, When to Say Yes and When to Say No To Take Control of Your Life* (Grand Rapids, MI: Zondervan Publishing House, 1992), p. 43.
8. *Ibid.*, pp. 241-246.
9. Cf. Lk 23:34.
10. Cloud and Townsend, *op. cit.*, pp. 245-246.

4

TO FORGIVE IS DIVINE

Forgiveness and Reconciliation

"Let all bitterness, anger, wrath, loud shouting, and slander be put away from you, along with all malice. Be kind to one another, compassionate, forgiving each other just as God forgave you in Christ." (Eph 4:31-32)

Stop! Before you skip over this section, *all of us* need to forgive and/or to be forgiven. Forgiving is all about getting rid of all anger and resentment in order to allow healing to take place. These are just some of the questions that I had to ask myself in this regard: Are you angry with your mother for developing this illness and dying on you? Are you angry with God for giving mom this terminal illness? Are you angry with yourself for not loving your mother more in the time that you had together? Who do you need to forgive or be forgiven by?

WHAT IS RESENTMENT?

Resentment is a common reaction we have when someone hurts us. How can that person hurt *me*? This resentment painfully manifests itself each time the memory of the person, hurt, or incident comes to mind. We cannot let the hurt go.

We tend to hold on to certain resentments towards others. We are often held in the grip of hurt and resentment, and the person responsible may not even be aware that he or she has this effect on us. In many cases, the person is long gone or even deceased.

Do you need to forgive? Consider this scenario.

Julie is a twenty-eight-year-old professional. She and her mother Sara have been estranged for over eight years, ever since Julie left the house to live with a 45-year-old accountant named Bill, whom she has since married against her father's very strong wishes.

Julie lives 200 miles from her mom and has not talked to or visited her during that time, and had decided not to do so while her mother lived with "that man," her father. But now that her mom has been diagnosed with a terminal illness, Julie feels the need to be with her. Julie just cannot forgive herself for staying away so long. Why wasn't she a better daughter to her mom when she had the chance?

Julie is angry with her father because he spent the greater part of the last twenty years drinking and physically abusing her mother, Sara. Julie bitterly recalls how he also physically and sexually abused her and in fact, that is why Julie left the house eight years ago. Now he won't even help out in her mom's care. He just sits in front of the TV and drinks vodka all day. The hospice nurse said that he was working out feelings of guilt for mistreating Sara so long. The nurse has arranged for a social worker to speak with and work with him.

Julie, an active member of St. Lucy's parish and an Extraordinary Minister of the Eucharist, has decided not to go to church anymore. How could such a loving God cause her mother to suffer like this? What kind of God can He be? How can she ever return to church again after what He has allowed to happen to her mother?

As you can see, there are many issues of anger and resentment in this family. We have not even addressed the resentment that Sara holds for each of these and her need for reconciliation before she dies. This is of great importance but cannot be discussed adequately here. A good resource book to read regarding the importance of closure and reconciliation before one dies is *Final Gifts* by Callanan and Kelley, hospice nurses.[1]

WHY DO WE NEED TO FORGIVE?

We forgive because as Christians we are obliged to do so! St. Paul tells us, "So then, as God's chosen ones, holy and beloved, clothe yourselves with heartfelt compassion, kindness, humility, gentleness, and patience; bear with one another and forgive one another, if one has a grievance against someone else. Just as the Lord forgave you, you too should do the same."[2] In the same way, when we say the *Our Father*, we pray "forgive us our trespasses as we forgive those who trespass against us."

That's a mighty powerful request of God. When you ask God to forgive you in this way, do you really know what you are asking Him? Do you *really* want Him to forgive you the same way you forgive others? Think about it. Is there anyone in your life whom you haven't forgiven? Think harder. The dying loved one? God? A family member? A friend? Yourself? If there is only one person we haven't forgiven, we are in effect asking God not to forgive us. Fortunately for us, God forgives unconditionally.

Another reason for forgiving is that if we don't forgive, we are condemned to carry the resentment and guilt around with us for years. This can lead to many physical and emotional problems down the road. An unforgiving heart is a heart not completely filled with love. If our hearts are not filled with love, how can we be receptive to the unconditional love that God has for us?

I received an e-mail message from a friend with this story from an anonymous author to help illustrate my point:

> One of my teachers had each of us bring a clear plastic bag and a sack of potatoes to school one day. For every person we had refused to forgive in our life, we were told to choose a potato, write on it the name and date, and put it in the plastic bag. Some of our bags, as you can imagine, were quite heavy.
>
> We were then told to carry this bag with us everywhere we went for one week, putting it beside our bed at night, on the car seat when driving, next to our desk at school. The hassle of lugging this around with us made it clear what a weight we were carrying spiritually, and how we had to pay attention to it all the time in order not to forget and leave it in embarrassing places.
>
> Naturally, the condition of the potatoes deteriorated to a nasty slime. This was a great metaphor for the price we pay for keeping our grudges and refusing to forgive! Too often we think of forgiveness as a gift to the other person, when it clearly is a gift for ourselves!
>
> So the next time you decide you can't forgive someone, ask yourself.... Isn't your bag heavy enough?

This little story graphically illustrates why we need to forgive. Without forgiveness, we carry around a sack of "slimy" resentment, pain, and negativity. It is clearly a load we do not need to be burdened with, especially when a loved one is dying.

FORGIVENESS VS. RECONCILIATION

Forgiving an injury does not condone or approve it. It means trying to let go of the hurt and not holding it against the person who offended us in the first place. After a conscious decision has been made to forgive someone, we *may* still continue to recall the situation or the offense and harbor a distaste for the one who hurt us. Forgiveness is therefore a decision of the will, and not a matter of feelings.[3] We have to make a conscious effort to forgive. It is an ongoing process and it won't happen overnight. It takes time and patience and much prayer. This is particularly true if it the hurt runs deep. It may even require a conscious decision to forgive *each time* the hurt surfaces. This is okay, as long as we are consciously deciding to forgive that person here and now.

Doesn't "she" have to apologize too?

No, not necessarily. Forgiveness comes from your heart. You release the chains of resentment that bound that person in your heart. It makes you feel better and you have accomplished what you should be doing as a Christian. The person may or may not ever know that you forgave them. At least not in this life.

Two-way forgiveness is known as *reconciliation* or mutual forgiveness. You forgive the person and they forgive you or at least apologize for the wrong they did. This does not mean that you have to be "best buddies" with that person in the future, or indeed that you have to have any relationship at all. As Christians we are reminded to work toward reconciliation: "Therefore, if you're presenting your offering at the altar and remember there that your brother has something against you, leave your offering there at the altar and first go and be reconciled with your brother, and then come and offer your gift."[4]

How can we tell that we are really forgiving someone? According to Fr. Tobin, author of *How to Forgive Yourself and Others,* the signs that true forgiveness has occurred are that we can pray for the person, sincerely wish them well, and if needed, help him or her in a needful situation.[5] It is difficult to be angry or resentful toward anyone that we are asking God to bless.

As mentioned above, we must forgive but do not then have to continue in a relationship with the person if we do not so desire. This would depend on what type of relationship there was with the person prior to the forgiveness, and whether we wish to continue or improve the relationship.

According to Fr. Tobin, the forgiveness process must be viewed in the light of these ten reminders[6]:

♦ To err is human, to forgive divine. The usual way we deal with hurt is through resentment and/or revenge. God's way is unconditional forgiveness.

♦ Forgiveness only occurs when we truly desire it.

♦ Failure to forgive usually involves our desire not to forgive.

♦ Forgiveness takes time and patience.

♦ We do not normally hurt others because we are evil or malicious. It is usually because we are weak and blind to the needs of others.

♦ There is a difference between the forgiveness of a hurt and the healing of a hurt. Forgiveness is an act of will. Healing takes time.

♦ There is a difference between forgiveness and reconciliation. Forgiveness takes only one person. Reconciliation requires two.

- Sometimes we have a hard time forgiving others because we cannot forgive ourselves. If we can't accept forgiveness from God and others, how can we possibly expect to forgive?
- Total healing may require professional help, especially in cases of abuse, etc.
- We must identify any feelings associated with the hurt before we can pray about it.

HOW DOES ONE FORGIVE?

Identify your feelings regarding the offense or wrongdoing. Ask yourself what is actually hurting you and why, or what you may have done to offend others. Make a list if need be and work through all of the issues.

Make a conscious decision to forgive the person who hurt you, or to apologize for the hurts you caused others. This may be very difficult. You may not want to forgive the person at first. Pray that you will someday be able to have the desire to forgive or to apologize to that person.

Write a letter to the individual stating that you would like to forgive him or her but you are having a hard time doing so, or that you desire their forgiveness. You can mail the letter if you wish, as long as in doing so you don't place yourself in physical danger or threat of abuse.

The person may be long gone or even deceased. In such a case, mentally forgive or apologize to that person in your heart with God as your witness. As Christians, we believe in the communion of saints and that we can communicate with the saints in heaven at any time. Let the person know in prayer that you have forgiven him or her and/or that you request their forgiveness. Let God do the rest.

If possible, and if it does not place you in undue danger or threat of abuse, tell the person that you forgive or that you ask forgiveness for yourself. Do not expect that the other person will care or be grateful, or that the other person desires to forgive you. He or she may even become more angry or detached. But at least you have offered your forgiveness and expressed your sorrow or regret.

Whenever the same hurt pops up, make a conscious effort to forgive again. Say a prayer for the person; pray for the strength to continue to be forgiving and for healing. Remember that total healing takes a desire to forgive, plus time and patience.

What happens if the person you resent is God?

Prayer, lots of prayer. The prayer that I find most effective is called experiential prayer. This is described in the chapter on prayer. It involves praying your daily experiences, good and bad. You can do it silently and mentally, or you can keep a journal. A typical journal entry for experiential prayer might read:

> "God, today I was very angry with you. Why did you allow me to be ridiculed by my co-workers? You know how I despise embarrassment. How could you do that to me? I know you love me and that everything that happens is part of a greater plan for my eternal happiness. Lord, please forgive me for doubting you. I love you, Lord."

A good resource for this type of prayer is *Praying Our Experiences,* by Joseph F. Schmidt, Saint Mary's Press.

Is it a sin to be angry with the Lord? No, of course not, as long as you don't turn your back on Him. He already knows all your thoughts before you do. In fact He enjoys your taking the time to dialogue with Him, and that you recognize and accept His will for you. Catholics have a wonderful sacrament for making peace with God. It is the Sacrament of Reconciliation. God loves and forgives unconditionally. Visit the confessional often.

Recall what Jesus asked His Father as He was dying on the cross, "Father, forgive them, they know not what they do."[7]

Notes

[1] Maggie Callanan and Patricia Kelley, *Final Gifts: Understanding the Special Awareness, Needs and Communications of the Dying* (NY: Bantam Books, 1997), p. 40.

[2] Col 3:12-13.

[3] Eamon Tobin, *How to Forgive Yourself and Others* (Liguori, MO: Liguori Press, 1993), p. 13.

[4] Mt 5:23-24.

[5] Tobin, *op. cit.*, p. 14.

[6] *Ibid.*, pp. 17-22.

[7] Lk 23:34.

5

BE NOT AFRAID!

Ethical Decisions: Prolong Life or Allow to Die?

"You shall not kill."
(Ex 20:13)

Hyperalimentation, computerized tomography scanners, micro-surgery, pulmonary artery catheterization, magnetic resonance imaging, electroencephalographs, pulmonary intubation and ventilation, and dopamine drips. These are only a fraction of the modes of therapies, tests and/or procedures used by medical personnel in modern healthcare facilities today. These and other therapies are used to save and hopefully prolong the lives of patients. Nothing is too advanced or costly to medical personnel in their pursuit to save lives. I know from first hand experience as a critical care nurse for ten years, that there is nothing more satisfying to medical professionals than to be able to save the life of someone who is entrusted to your care.

Sometimes those patients who are saved lead high quality lives as a result of these miraculous saving therapies. Many times, however, well-intentioned medical personnel will extend the life of a terminally ill patient only to prolong the suffering and grief of both the patient and the family.

Occasionally it is better to discontinue advanced medical care, or not to start it at all. In the effort to preserve human dignity, difficult choices regarding the initiation and/or the continuance of advanced life support must frequently be made. What does the Church have to say about all this? What is its official teaching regarding:

- ♦ Excessively burdensome means of prolonging or sustaining life or health
- ♦ Withholding or withdrawal of excessively burdensome means of prolonging or sustaining life or health
- ♦ Resuscitation/Do Not Resuscitate Orders
- ♦ Euthanasia/Assisted Suicide
- ♦ Advanced Directives (Living Wills and Durable Power of Attorney for Health Care)
- ♦ Autopsies/Organ Donation
- ♦ Cremation/Christian Burial

Each of these topics will be discussed below from the point of view of medical ethics and ecclesiastical teaching.

RESPECT FOR HUMAN LIFE

For the Roman Catholic Church, human life is a *gift* from God, a gift of which we are the stewards and not the master.
"Human life is sacred because from the beginning it involves the creative action of God and it remains forever in a special relationship with the Creator, who is its sole end. God alone is the Lord of life from its beginning until its end: no one can under any circumstance claim for himself the right directly to destroy an innocent human being."[1]

The principles taught by the Church on end of life decisions express this regard for the dignity of human life. "By taking on our human nature, that is, by fully sharing our life, the eternal Son of God taught us how precious each human life really is in His Father's eyes."[2] The Church offers the following moral principles as a guide to the faithful in making decisions regarding medical care and treatment for the sick and dying[3]:

♦ Our most basic God-given right is the right to life.
♦ We do not have the right to take our own lives, nor directly to bring about the death of any innocent person.
♦ Christian faith reveals the true meaning of suffering.
♦ Each of us is obliged to care for the gift of life and health that God has given us.
♦ No patient is obliged to accept or demand useless medical interventions.
♦ There is no moral obligation to employ useful but excessively burdensome medical interventions; however, the meaning of "excessively burdensome" must be properly understood.

Death is a natural process that can lead to the fullness of eternal life. The Catholic tradition holds that all persons have a serious responsibility to preserve their lives and health, but that *excessively burdensome means* to do so are not morally required.[4]

EXCESSIVELY BURDENSOME VS. NOT EXCESSIVELY BURDENSOME MEANS OF PROLONGING/SUSTAINING LIFE AND HEALTH

Ethically speaking, excessively burdensome measures of care are those that place undue physical, mental, financial, or spiritual burden on the patient or family.[5] Those which do not cause serious physical, mental, financial or spiritual strain on the patient or the family are considered not excessively burdensome. Burdens vary and are determined in each individual circumstance or situation. The question to be answered in each case is whether the benefit to the patient justifies the burden it imposes.

Healthcare personnel and theologians do not always agree on the same definition of excessively burdensome means of therapy. Medical personnel may consider some excessively burdensome care standard treatment because of its ease of administration and/or use. The same treatment might be considered futile and/or excessively burdensome to some patients in certain circumstances, elevating the therapy to an excessively burdensome measure.[6]

It is by now obvious that there can be no general statement of principles that can be used in every situation and circumstance. It is wise to say that the virtue of *prudence* is called for here. In making these decisions, it is vital to draw on our personal moral instruction and experience, along with the advice of medical personnel and the clergy. "Whether a given treatment is necessary or useful to a particular patient is a medical question requiring the expertise of health care professionals. Whether a particular treatment is excessively burdensome to an individual patient is a moral question requiring the advice of a priest or someone else well trained in sound moral theology."[7] Patients and their families should seek the advice and guidance of the Church when making decisions of a moral nature.

The statement that can be conclusively made is that although patients may morally decide that a particular mode of therapy is excessively burdensome, they may never decide that their lives are so useless or burdensome as to refuse the ordinary medical treatments needed to sustain life. The moral judgment to be made is whether the benefits received from a proposed treatment justify the difficulties, suffering, and expense required of a patient and family.

Terminal Illness

Special consideration is needed for those who are terminally ill and whose death is imminent despite advances in modern science. The Commission for Catholic Life Issues (1992), of the Archdiocese of Los Angeles states, "Treatments that are usually regarded as 'life-sustaining' are not so in this circumstance and are therefore not morally required, unless the person is not spiritually prepared for death and the treatment might prolong life enough to enable him or her to receive the sacraments or fulfill other moral duties (e.g., update a will, reconcile a hurt friendship, etc.)."[8] In the absence of such duties and when the person is spiritually prepared for death, it is often considered appropriate to withdraw excessive or burdensome modes of therapy to make the last hours or days of a dying person more pleasant, dignified, and peaceful, even if the act would seem to quicken death.

To Withhold or Withdraw Excessively Burdensome Therapy

There is no moral difference between withholding of a treatment and withdrawing the treatment once started, if the treatment is clearly "excessively burdensome." The problem that generally arises is the emotional attachment. Once a treatment is started, it is emotionally more difficult to stop it, even though one is well aware that there is a moral right to do so. In these cases it might be the more prudent decision not to start treatment at all if it seems clear that it will have to be discontinued at a later point.

The dilemma of whether or not a treatment will later turn out to be useful or burdensome can arise. In these situations, it is better to opt for the therapy. If at a later date it becomes obvious that the therapy is indeed futile or extraordinary, a decision to discontinue it at that time can be made with good conscience.[9]

Resuscitate vs. Do Not Resuscitate Orders

Resuscitation generally applies to a life saving procedure known as Cardiopulmonary Resuscitation (CPR). This is an act by which a lone rescuer or a team of rescuers attempts to maintain cardiac (heart) circulation and ventilation (breathing) throughout the body when a patient clinically dies, i.e., his heart and breathing stops. This is done using a ratio of chest compressions to mouth-to-mouth breaths.

CPR has varying degrees of success depending on the type of death the person has endured, the performance of the rescuers, the body chemistry levels, and a slew of other various factors. It does frequently come with a price. Even if done correctly, CPR can fracture ribs, lacerate the liver, and/or puncture the vital organs. If a rescuer waits too long to initiate CPR, the patient can develop brain damage. The medical community considers these minor complications when compared to the possibility of "bringing back" from the clutches of death someone who has clinically died. Unless otherwise specified, all patients in health care institutions are required to have CPR initiated if they go into cardiac arrest.

However, a health care provider can give a *Do Not Resuscitate* (DNR) order based on the patient's condition/prognosis, a lucid patient's desires, or by instructions set forth in *advanced directives* (discussed below). If a family or patient decides against resuscitation in case of death, the same prudence used to determine withholding or withdrawing excessively burdensome means of care needs to be applied.

In the case of a Catholic, this resuscitative effort can buy the person a little more time to receive the sacraments or make peace with a family member. Even if CPR is considered futile or burdensome in the case of a terminally ill individual, it can be spiritually life saving in such cases.[10]

EUTHANASIA AND SUICIDE

It is prohibited by the Church and the laws of God to practice *euthanasia* or to commit *suicide*. The word "euthanasia" comes from the Greek word *euthanatos,* which means "easy death." A distinction must be made between direct and indirect (or passive) euthanasia.

Direct euthanasia (traditionally referred to as *"mercy killing"*) is a deliberate act that brings about the death of another in order to alleviate that person's suffering. Direct euthanasia is always morally wrong, no matter how noble the motive. An example of this would be the administering of a lethal injection to someone who was in intractable pain.

Indirect (or passive) euthanasia is deliberately allowing a person who is in imminent danger of death to die rather than to intervene to save the life of that individual when there is a reasonable prognosis of a good outcome should such intervention take place.

The Congregation for the Doctrine of the Faith (CDF) in its *Declaration on Euthanasia* describes *euthanasia* as the intentional ending of the life of another, whether by commission or omission, in order to relieve suffering.

Suicide is the intentional ending of one's own life. *Assisted Suicide* is helping another to end his or her life by a deliberate act of commission or omission.[11] Both are objectively wrong as they usurp God's sovereignty over human life.[12]

If both of these are objectively wrong, wouldn't withholding or withdrawing treatment constitute active euthanasia or assisted suicide? The answer to that question is emphatically, "No!" There is a profound difference between allowing someone to die and the intentional causing of death through commission or omission. This difference is not defined by the outcome — the death of the patient — but by the intent of the person causing or allowing the death. If the individual causing the death has made a willful decision to take another's life to alleviate that person's suffering, then it would be considered euthanasia; if he or she were asked to do so by the one who was suffering, it would be considered assisted suicide — in most states, murder.

The CDF *Declaration on Euthanasia* states: "Such a refusal (of life-sustaining treatment) is not the equivalent of suicide; on the contrary, it should be considered as an acceptance of the human condition, or a wish to avoid the application of a medical procedure disproportionate to the results that can be expected, or a desire not to impose excessive expense on the family or the community."[13]

In *Evangelium Vitae*, Pope John Paul II states: "Certainly there is an obligation to care for oneself and to allow oneself to be cared for, but this duty must take account of concrete circumstances. It needs to be determined whether the means of treatment available are objectively proportionate to the prospects for improvement."[14]

What determines whether withholding or withdrawing treatment is morally right or wrong? The answer lies in distinguishing between excessively burdensome and not excessively burdensome means of preserving life and health.

ADVANCED DIRECTIVES (LIVING WILLS AND DPAHC)

Advanced directives are methods by which a person gives instructions regarding his future health care decisions when he is unable to do so due to physical incapacitation or psychological incompetence.

Although the laws vary from state to state, there are generally three types of advanced directives[15]:

◆ *Durable Power of Attorney for Health Care (DPAHC)* is a written document appointing a health care agent who, with or without written instructions, will act for the patient when he or she is unable to do so;

◆ *Living Wills* are written instructions authorizing in advance the administration, withholding, or withdrawal of life-sustaining procedures if the person is in a terminal condition with death imminent or in a persistent vegetative state;

◆ *Oral statements* may be made to health care providers in the presence of a witness leaving instructions involving life-sustaining care or the appointment of an agent.

In preparing advanced directives, one should follow these guidelines and perhaps speak to a pastor, priest, or deacon as well as a medical professional.[16]

◆ Blanket statements and instructions should be avoided. You should not state that you wish to reject certain therapies under "all" circumstances, or state without qualification what types of therapy you want restricted. For instance, a person instructs in a living will that he wishes no CPR started upon clinical death, when in reality CPR could be a simple procedure to save his or her life after an automobile accident. In another situation, a person may ask to withhold medical treatment without being aware that most hospitals and courts consider food and water a medical treatment. By rejecting food and water, one can die of starvation and dehydration. The Church generally views food and water as being *not excessively burdensome* means of therapy and withdrawal of such is usually forbidden (unless nutrients can no longer be assimilated or their use is determined to be excessively burdensome or dangerous).

♦ Choose a health care agent who has a character similar to your own who can make good judgments in your behalf in difficult situations.

♦ Appoint someone whom you can trust to follow the teachings of the Church. Do not choose anyone who disagrees with or would be expected to go against the teachings of the Church.

♦ Choose someone who will be available for your care in the distant future. It probably would not be prudent to choose as an agent someone who is a military member and who will be expected to change duty stations several times in the future, or an individual who is significantly older than you who may not outlive you.

♦ Make sure your agent completely understands your desires in your health care instructions.

♦ There should be a statement that these directives apply if and only if death is imminent. The Church only allows refusal when the treatment is considered futile or would present a burdensome prolongation of life.

♦ Review your advanced directives periodically with your agent, clergy, and doctor.

♦ Make copies and distribute them to the above people.

Autopsies/Organ Donation

According to the *Catechism of the Catholic Church*, "Autopsies can be morally permitted for legal inquests or scientific research. The free gift of organs after death is legitimate and can be meritorious."[17] Note here that organ donation is a "free-will gift" and cannot be forced upon or taken from one without their consent. Note also that the sale of organs raises some serious ethical and legal questions. The operative phrase is "free gift"; to profit from such a gift is wrong and generally illegal everywhere in the world.

Christian Burial and/or Cremation

The Catholic Church no longer requires a deceased member of the faithful to be buried in sacred (consecrated) soil, but it is recommended. Along the same lines, cremation is no longer prohibited if the remains are disposed of properly. If ashes are to be buried at sea, they must not be sprinkled, but buried intact.

Canon Law states: "The Church earnestly recommends that the pious custom of burial be retained; but it does not forbid cremation, unless this is chosen for reasons which are contrary to Christian teaching."[18] These reasons would include denying or rejecting a belief in the resurrection of the body at the end of time.

Check your home diocese to learn of any special norms or guidelines. As of this printing, the Archdiocese of Washington, D.C. has published the following policy in regards to ashes and funeral Masses: "(If) the person is cremated immediately after death, there is no celebration of a vigil or Funeral Mass. A Mass for the Dead, however, may certainly be celebrated at a convenient time for the family. In this case, the cremated remains are not to be present. The rite of committal, however, may be celebrated when the ashes of the deceased are interred or buried."[19]

Notes

1   Cf. *Catechism of the Catholic Church* (CCC), §2258; CDF, instruction, *Donum Vitae,* intro. 5.
2   "Care of the Sick and Dying." Maryland Catholic Conference of Bishops, Task Force on Medical Decisions, October 1993, p. 4.
3   Cf. "Nutrition and Hydration: Moral Pastoral Reflections," NCCB Committee on Pro-Life Activities, April 1992, pp. 3-6.
4   David Bohr, *Catholic Moral Tradition.* 2nd ed. (Huntington, IN: Our Sunday Visitor Press, 1999), p. 311.
5   *Ibid.*
6   "Moral Issues Regarding Advance Healthcare Directives and Living Wills," Commission for Catholic Life Issues (Los Angeles, CA/Princeton, NJ: Scepter Booklets, 1992), p. 14.
7   "Care of the Sick and Dying," p. 10.
8   "Moral Issues Regarding Advance Healthcare Directives and Living Wills," p. 22.
9   *Ibid.*, p. 16.
10 *Ibid.*, p. 19.
11 *Declaration on Euthanasia,* Congregation for the Doctrine of Faith, 1980, p. 514.
12 "Moral Issues Regarding Advance Healthcare Directives and Living Wills," p. 19.
13 *Declaration on Euthanasia,* p. 514.
14 John Paul II, Encyclical Letter, *Evangelium Vitae,* The Gospel of Life (March 25, 1995), no. 65.
15 "Care of the Sick and Dying," pp. 21-22.
16 *Ibid.*, pp. 25-27.
17 CCC, 2300.
18 CIC, Can. 1176, §3; CCC, 2301.
19 *Sacramental Norms and Guidelines,* Archdiocese of Washington, DC, p. 89.

6

PREPARATION FOR THE FINAL JOURNEY
The Last Things

"Then the angel showed me the river of the water of life. It sparkled like crystal, flowing from the throne of God and the Lamb."
(Rv 22:1)

The Four Last Things

Life is short and death is sure.
The hour of death remains obscure.

A soul you have and only one,
If that be lost all hope is gone.

Waste not time, while time shall last;
For after death 'tis ever past.

All-seeing God, your Judge will be,
And heaven or hell your destiny.

All earthly things will speed away,
Eternity, alone, will stay.[1]

We must all prepare ourselves for the "last things," death, judgment, hell, and heaven. Death is inevitable. St. Augustine said that "Everything in life, good or bad, is uncertain, except death. Only death is certain." We start dying as soon as we are born.

We all face personal judgment with Jesus and all mankind

together will be judged at the end of time. Personal judgment happens when we die. In the letter to the Hebrews, we are told, "It has been ordained that human beings die once and then are judged."[2] According to the Catholic Church, "Those who die in God's grace and friendship and are perfectly purified live forever with Christ."[3] Those who die in God's grace and friendship, but are still imperfect, are assured salvation but must achieve purification and holiness at a way station we call purgatory. In *Fire of Love, Understanding Purgatory,* St. Catherine of Genoa tells us: "Thus a great happiness is granted them (the souls in purgatory) that never fails; rather it grows as they draw nearer to God.... For every glimpse that can be had of God exceeds any pain or joy a man can feel."[4]

Unless we use our free will to choose God, we cannot be united with Him in heaven. These poor souls who die separated from the Love of God enter a state of "definitive self-exclusion" from communion with God known as "hell."[6] St Catherine of Genoa again teaches that hell is a place whose inhabitants are fully aware of the existence of God, but never see Him. "Thus are the souls of the damned from whom has been taken any hope of ever seeing their bread, which is God the true Savior."[7]

That is why it is important that our loved ones be reconciled with God before they die. If they lived a life in God's grace and friendship, they are just about there. It is never wasted effort to reconcile with Jesus one more time.

MINISTERING THE SACRAMENTS TO THE SICK

This is what used to be known (and sometimes still is for us old timers) as the "Last Rites." The whole package generally includes the following:

- ◆ The Sacrament of Reconciliation
- ◆ The Sacrament of the Eucharist and Viaticum
- ◆ The Anointing of the Sick

The first and most important issue to be mentioned is that you do not need to be on your deathbed to receive these sacraments. As soon as "anyone of the faithful begins to be in danger of death from sickness or old age, the fitting time for him to receive this sacrament has certainly already arrived."[8] If a sick person who has received this anointing recovers or temporarily becomes well, he can in the case of another grave illness receive the sacrament again. If a person's health deteriorates during the period of the same illness, he may also receive it again.[9] Each of the sacraments is discussed below.

SACRAMENTS OF INITIATION

These three sacraments, Baptism, Confirmation, and Holy Eucharist are known as the *Sacraments of Initiation* into the Body of Christ. For the faithful born into the Catholic faith, these are received over time. Baptism is required before any other sacrament can be administered. Though these three sacraments are not classified among those used in ministering to the sick, they may very well, on occasion, be necessary if they have not already been received. Those who have not been baptized and confirmed and who have not yet received their First Holy Communion and are in imminent danger of dying may receive all three sacraments at one time.

Sacrament of Baptism

Baptized Christians are members of the Body of Christ and adopted children of God.[10] Having died to sin, they are part of the "community" of the Church, having obtained the graces needed to be a Christian in good standing.

Sacrament of Confirmation

"Confirmation is the sacrament by which those born anew in baptism receive the seal of the Holy Spirit, the Gift of the Father."[11] We get an increase of the gifts of the Holy Spirit in this sacrament and special strength in order to fuel our lifetime witness to Christ and service to others.[12]

Sacrament of Holy Eucharist

In the Eucharist we are strengthened and supported. Jesus Himself is truly present in the sacred host and precious blood. Imagine receiving the body, blood, soul and divinity of Our Lord Jesus Christ every time we receive Holy Communion, the same body that was present at Calvary and is present now in heaven and in all the tabernacles of the world. He who suffered on the Cross for us is present now in our suffering.

Jesus said, "Amen, amen, I say to you, unless you eat the flesh of the Son of Man and drink his blood, you do not have life within you. Whoever feeds on my flesh and drinks my blood has eternal life, and I will raise him up on the last day. For my flesh is true food, and my blood is true drink. Whoever feeds on my flesh and drinks my blood remains in me and I in him. Just as the living Father sent me, and I live because of the Father, so too the one who feeds on me will live because of me."[13]

What better "food" to give a sick loved one than the Body and Blood of Our Lord? Think of the healing properties it has.

The woman with a hemorrhage just touched the tassel of Jesus' cloak, and she was cured.[14]

Conditions For Receiving Holy Communion

The communicant must be in unity with the faithful of the Catholic Church and be in a state of grace, free from all deadly sin. In the case of the sick and aged *and those who care for them*, the mandated fast of one hour from food and drink (except water and medicines) is waived.

Viaticum

For those whose death is imminent, the Church offers the Eucharist as *viaticum*. This is Holy Communion received by those preparing for their final journey, their *passing over* to the Father. "The sacrament of Christ once dead and now risen, the Eucharist, is here the sacrament of passing over from death to life, from this world to the Father."[15]

SACRAMENTS OF HEALING

The sacraments of Reconciliation and Anointing of the Sick are called the *Sacraments of Healing*.

Sacrament of Reconciliation

It is through the sacrament of Penance or Reconciliation that the baptized can be reconciled with God and with the Church. Reconciliation brings us God's healing and forgiveness for sins committed after the sacrament of Baptism. What an exhilarating experience for all who worthily receive this sacrament. It gives peace to the dying, knowing that their sins are forgiven and that they may die in peace.

Requirements for Reconciliation

According to the Church's command "after having attained the age of discretion, each of the faithful is bound by an obligation faithfully to confess serious sins at least once a year" (CIC, canon 989). It is recommended, however, that the sacrament of Reconciliation be received frequently during the year in order to "form our conscience, fight against evil tendencies, let ourselves be healed by Christ and progress in the life of the Spirit."[16] It is certainly appropriate for the sick and dying.

Sacrament of Anointing of the Sick

"Is anyone among you suffering under adversity? He should pray! Is anyone cheerful? He should sing songs of praise. Is anyone among you sick? He should call the elders of the church and have them pray over him and anoint him with oil in the name of the Lord — prayer rooted in faith will save whoever is ill and the Lord will raise him up. And even if he has sinned, the Lord will forgive him."[17] In a serious illness, we experience our human mortality. We come face to face with the reality that we are going to die.

Through this sacrament, God communes with us as we prepare for our final meeting with Him. The entire Church asks God to lighten our sufferings, forgive us our sins, and bring us to everlasting life with Him and all the hosts of heaven.[18]

One need not be in the final moments of life to receive this sacrament. By its very nature its purpose is to restore health of body, mind and soul.[19] As discussed in Chapter One, this sacrament helps us to share more fully in the cross of Christ.[20]

By the special grace of the Anointing of the Sick, the following effects are obtained:

♦ the uniting of the suffering of the sick person to the passion and suffering of Christ for the person's own good and for the good of the whole Church

♦ strengthening, peace, and courage to endure the suffering of illness or old age

♦ the forgiveness of sins if not obtained in the sacrament of Reconciliation

♦ the restoration of health, if it is God's will and conducive to the salvation of the person's soul

♦ the preparation for passing over to life eternal.[21]

WILL OUR LOVED ONE BE PREPARED FOR ETERNITY?

Spiritual care is every bit as important as medical and emotional care, and as any healthcare provider will tell you, holistic healing must encompass the "whole" person: physically, emotionally, and spiritually. The Church officially teaches that our life as Christians is lived in preparation for the four "last things": death, judgment, heaven, and hell. .

It is important for all Christians to reconcile with God before they die. As a caregiver, you must try to assure that the soul of your loved one is spiritually ready for death in the event that he is not capable to do so without assistance. For Catholics, this means reconciliation with God through the reception of the sacraments, especially the sacraments of Reconciliation, Holy Eucharist and the Anointing of the Sick.

Notes

[1] Charles Carty and Leslie Rumble, *Why Squander Illness: Prayers and Thoughts for Catholic and Non-Catholic Patients* (Rockford, IL: Tan Books and Publishers, Inc., 1974), p. 33.

[2] Heb 9:27.

[3] CCC, 1023.

[4] Ibid., 1030.

[5] St. Catherine of Genoa, *Fire of Love, Understanding Purgatory* (Manchester, NH: Sophia Institute Press, 1996), p. 84.

[6] CCC, 1033.

[7] *Fire of Love,* p. 41.

[8] Second Vatican Council, The Constitution on the Sacred Liturgy, *Sacrosanctum Concilium,* 73; cf. CIC cc. 1004 §1; 1005; 1007.

[9] CCC, 1514-1515.

[10] *Ibid.,* 1266.

[11] *Handbook for Today's Catholic* (Liguori, MO: Liguori Publications, 1994).

[12] CCC, 1302-1303.

[13] Jn 6:54-57.

[14] Cf. Mt 9:20-22.

[15] CCC, 1524; Cf. Jn 13:1.

[16] CCC, 1458.

[17] Jm 5:13-16.

[18] CCC, 1520.

[19] *Ibid.,* 1514-1515.

[20] *Ibid.,* 1521.

[21] *Ibid.,* 1532.

7

PERSEVERANCE IN PRAYER
The Power of Prayer

*"Pray constantly, give thanks no matter what happens,
for this is God's will for you in Christ Jesus."*
(1 Th 5:17-18)

The Apostles knew the power of prayer. They asked Jesus to show them how to pray.[1] In response, Jesus told them how to pray to the Father.[2] He taught them perseverance in prayer through the parable of the 'midnight friend'[3] and the persistent woman.[4] He brought it home by explaining that prayer is private between the individual and God[5] and that a person should be humble in prayer.[6] Jesus told us that if we want something, all we have to do is ask. "Ask and it will be given to you; seek and you will find; knock and the door will be opened to you. For whoever asks, receives; whoever seeks, finds; and to whoever knocks, the door will be opened."[7] He taught them to never stop praying.[8]

WHY SHOULD I PRAY?

You may ask that question, especially in view of the fact that your loved one is dying. Isn't it too late? Why pray now? What possible good can it do?

Praying brings you closer to God. Prayer is a dialogue, a communion, between you and God. Ask God for a miracle; it may just happen. "Whatever you ask for in my name, I will do it, so that the Father may be glorified in the Son."[9] Praying helps us to find meaning in suffering. "Is anyone among you suffering under adversity? He should pray."[10] Prayer helps us to endure hardships. "Rejoice in your hope, bear up when you're afflicted, *persevere in prayer*."[11]

It is times like these when you need Jesus the most. Jesus tells us, "Come to me, all you who labor and are burdened, and I will give you rest. Take my yoke upon you and learn from me, for I am meek and humble of heart; and you will find rest for yourselves. For my yoke is easy, and my burden light."[12] What an invitation! Why do we not take advantage of it? "Therefore I say to you, whatever you ask for in prayer, believe that you have received it and it will be yours."[13]

Even if you are angry with Jesus for your loved one's getting a terminal illness, tell Him so. He already knows you are angry. He wants you to come to Him for comfort. "Your Father knows what you need before you ask him."[14] We are telling Jesus the experiences of our day. We are sharing the good and the bad. We are sharing the joyful and sad. We can thank Him for our gifts and for the trials He has given us. We are just conversing with Jesus.

DIVERSITY IN PRAYER

This section is not intended as a theology lesson. It is provided so that you may see the many types of prayer available to you for solace, comfort, and healing. The following paragraphs will discuss the forms of prayer and the different methods in which to pray.

Forms of Prayer

Adoration/Praise

According to the *Catechism of the Catholic Church*, this form of prayer acknowledges our status as creatures before God. It exalts His majesty and greatness and lauds God. It gives Him the Glory to which He is entitled. It recognizes God as God.[15]

Contrition

In this form of prayer we ask God to forgive the wrongs we have committed against Him and our neighbors. These wrongs can be those of which we are aware and those of which we are not aware. We pray prayers of contrition for our eternal well being and the well being of others.

Thanksgiving

The Church's celebration of the Eucharist is this type of prayer.[16] It shows our gratitude to God for His unconditional love for us and for all He has done for us and given us. We should be thankful for our trials as well as our joys, for in our suffering we are glorified with Him.[17]

Petition

This is the most common form of prayer because it is the most spontaneous. It is the prayer of the creature asking the Creator for help. This type of prayer is typified by the phrase, "There are no atheists in foxholes." Associated with this form of prayer is the prayer of intercession in which we ask the Lord for a favor on behalf of someone else.[18]

Methods of Praying

Community/Public Prayer

This is the most important of all prayers for the Church as it is the public worship of the people of God.[19] "Again I say to you, if two of you agree on earth about any matter they ask for, it shall be granted to them by my heavenly Father."[20] Public prayer takes a variety of forms.

The Mass

The Mass is the highest form of community prayer. "It is the whole community, the Body of Christ united with its Head, that celebrates."[21] Through Faith and ritual, while in union with the whole Church, both heavenly and visible, we join in the eternal celebration of that heavenly liturgy which is celebrated in the "new Jerusalem" on high. We do not have to wait to die to go to heaven, for the Mass is heaven on earth. "Those who even now celebrate it without signs are already in the heavenly liturgy, where celebration is wholly communion and feast."[22]

St. John Chrysostom in his *Treatise on the Priesthood* (circa 386 AD) asks us: "When you see the Lord immolated and lying upon the altar, and the priest bent over that sacrifice praying, and all the people empurpled by that precious blood, can you think that you are still among men and on earth? Or are you not lifted up to heaven?"

The Divine Office/Liturgy of the Hours

This is the "Church's Prayer" also known as Christian Prayer. It is prayed at specified hours of the day, generally by the ordained, religious, and those in community life. However, all are invited to pray the Liturgy of the Hours alone or in common.

Devotions: The Rosary and the Divine Mercy Chaplet

This form of prayer is the most popular form of community prayer for the average person and rightly so. Many miracles have been obtained through the power of the Rosary.

Personal Prayer

The Holy Eucharist

If prayer is a dialogue or communion with God, what better way to commune with God than through the Holy Eucharist, the Blessed Sacrament? The most intimate communion you can have with God this side of heaven is through the Eucharist, which is Jesus Christ, the Living God "yesterday, today and forever."

It is important for both the caregiver and the care receiver to receive sacraments on a regular basis if and when possible. The sacraments give us grace, which helps us to keep close to Jesus. Jesus will give us comfort and lighten our burden. The Eucharist especially should be received daily or as frequently as possible. If you cannot take your loved one to Mass, arrange for a priest, deacon, or extraordinary minister of the Eucharist to give Communion to your loved one. The criteria for the reception of Communion by the sick and their caregivers were discussed in Chapter 6.

Adoration of the Blessed Sacrament

For the patient who is ambulatory and for the caregiver, visits to the Blessed Sacrament are equally important, whether exposed for adoration or in the tabernacle. Jesus asks us, "Could you not keep watch for one hour?"[23] Jesus suffered for us. He wants us to find comfort in Him. What better comfort is there than knowing that we are in the presence of the Risen Christ, the creator of the universe?

Spontaneous Prayer

These are the prayers we pray from our heart every day, little prayers such as "God, please give me strength," "Thank you Lord, for a beautiful day," "Thank you, Lord, for my trials as well as my blessings for it is in trials that I grow in communion with you," "Lord, please heal my brother," or "What an awesome God you are, Lord."

Spontaneous prayer also includes *experiential prayer*. Experiential prayer is discussed more fully in the chapter on forgiveness.

Formal Prayer

These are the prayers that most of us memorized as a child, the "Our Father," "Hail Mary," etc. The Rosary and the Divine Mercy Chaplet when said in private are included in this category. A compendium of these prayers is found in Appendix B.

Meditative Prayer

This prayer is also known as *discursive meditation*. It is a method of private prayer which is centuries old and has been used extensively by monastics. It involves reading a section of Sacred Scripture, *Lectio Divina,* over and over. When a verse strikes you as being special, stop and meditate on it; then read the passage again keeping the insights from your reflection in mind. It is actually "praying Scripture." It is like reading a letter from a friend or relative. One reading is not enough. You have to go over and over the letter to find the "deeper meaning" behind the lines. This letter usually entrances us so much that we have to write a letter back to the writer.[24]

Centering Prayer

"But when you pray, go to your inner room, close the door, and pray to your Father in secret. And your Father who sees in secret will repay you."[25] Although I try to incorporate many forms of prayer throughout the day, this is by far my personal favorite. It is through this type of prayer that I can recline at Jesus' side, as the beloved disciple, and just listen to Him in awe.[26]

If *discursive meditation* is pondering a letter received from a loved one, than centering prayer is like sitting quietly at the side of a dear friend. Between good friends no words are necessary. "Heart speaks to heart without words." Just being in the company of each other speaks volumes.

Although it is not for everyone, I recommend that you try centering prayer if you feel called to do so. The procedure for centering prayer is outlined in Appendix C.

PERSEVERANCE IN PRAYER: A SUMMARY

It is important to pray and to commune with God, and it is especially helpful during times of trial and stress. It is when prayers may seem useless that we often need them the most.

The most perfect form of prayer and communion with God is to be found in the Holy Eucharist. "Those who receive the Eucharist are united more closely to Christ. Through it Christ unites them to all the faithful in one body, the Church."[27]

St. Leo the Great writes: "Our participation in the Body and Blood of Christ does nothing else except this: that we *pass over* into what we have received, into Christ; for we have died with Him and have been raised with Him. And thus we bear Him *within*, both in our spirit and in our flesh, at all times" (*Sermon* 63:7, 135-141).

Prayer can involve more than one form and is unique to each individual. Everyone should be comfortable with his or her own form of prayer and adapt it to his or her own situation in life.

We pray through the help of the Holy Spirit. Ask God to help you to enrich your personal prayer life. Ask Him to give you the graces of the Holy Spirit in prayer.

Notes

[1] Cf. Lk 11:1.
[2] Cf. Mt 6:9.
[3] Cf. Lk 11:5-13.
[4] Cf. Lk 18:1-8.
[5] Cf. Mt 6:6.
[6] Cf. Lk 18:9-14.
[7] Mt 7:7-8.
[8] Cf. Lk 18:1; 1 Th 5:17-18.
[9] Jn 14:13.
[10] Jm 5:13.
[11] Rm 12:12.
[12] Mt 11:28-30.
[13] Mk 11:24.
[14] Mt 6:8.
[15] CCC, 2628 and 2639.
[16] *Ibid.*, 2637.
[17] Cf. Rm 8:17.
[18] Cf. Jm 5:16.
[19] John Jay Hughes, *Centering Prayer: How to Pray From the Heart* (Liguori, MO: Liguori Publishing, 1981), p. 5.
[20] Mt 18:19.
[21] CCC, 1140.
[22] *Ibid.*, 1089; 1090; 1136.
[23] Mk 14:37b.
[24] Hughes, *Centering Prayer,* p. 9.
[25] Mt 6:6.
[26] Cf. Jn 13:23.
[27] CCC, 1396.

8

SAYING GOODBYE AND LETTING GO

Knowing When to Give Your Loved One Permission to Die

"We said farewell to one another... and they went back home."
(Acts 21:6)

You have it all figured out. You know the beauty and meaning in your loved one's suffering. You are appropriately dealing with the grieving process and helping others to do the same. You have forgiven God, yourself, and your loved one for getting this disease. You have prepared your loved one spiritually for death and now they are ready to *"go home."* Are you ready to let them go? Will you give them permission to go?

It may seem strange, even sadistic to tell someone that it is okay to die. But when your loved one is ready to die, they will most likely already know it. It is important for many dying individuals to be reassured that the family will be able to get along without them; they will want to know if it is okay to die.

How Do I Know My Loved One
Really Accepts Death and Is Ready to Die?

In the book *Final Gifts*, Callanan and Kelley, registered nurse team-members of hospice, beautifully discuss the phenomenon of "Nearing Death Awareness" (NDA) through a series of end

of life stories. NDA usually occurs in people dying of slowly progressive illnesses such as cancer, AIDS, or lung disease.[1] These
dying loved ones leave this world gradually, developing ties with
the new one (occasionally simultaneously).

There are those instances when your loved one appears to
be communicating with family members already departed, with
celestial creatures such as angels, or with Jesus or the Blessed Vir-
gin. They may be experiencing two realities simultaneously, the
reality of this world and that of the next. These people often de-
scribe the beauty of the next world in terms of colors, peace, or
the wonderfully warm and bright light that draws them closer
to it.

Our first inclination is to think that they are confused or
delusional or that they have become distant or detached. Often
they cannot explain the things they are experiencing, which only
compounds the doubt of those who do not share what they are
experiencing.

Final Gifts relates several of the documented thousands of
end of life stories indicating that this is a fairly common awareness that dying persons have just as they are preparing to die.

In their communication with these other beings, the dying
person may be subtly requesting permission to die. They may not
want to leave this world until they know that it is okay with you
or with other special family members or friends to die. They may
say, "They are coming for me," or something similar.

How Do I Give My Loved One
Permission to *"Go Home"*?

When it is time, your loved ones will let you know in some way.
Talk to them. Listen to their clues. Discuss these with your family
members and support system.

When it has been ascertained that your loved one is ready to die, you might say something like,

> "Mother, we/I know that you are ready to leave us. We/I have all talked it over and although we/I will miss you, we are ready to let you go. We/I hope to see you soon and know that you will help to prepare a place for us/me. You can go home whenever you are ready. We/I love you."

You will in all probability discover that your loved one will die more peacefully knowing that you will be okay and that it is permissible for them to leave. In fact, the end might then come sooner then you anticipated. All persons involved will be more at ease when the decision is made to say goodbye and let go.

WHAT IS PREVENTING ME FROM SAYING GOODBYE?

There are probably as many reasons as there are individuals. Death is a private event; we are born alone and we die alone. A segment of a song from the popular rock opera *Jesus Christ Superstar* makes the point, "to conquer death, you only have to die."

The most obvious reason why we find ourselves unable to say goodbye is that we will miss the loved one dearly. A piece of us will leave with them. We wonder if we will ever see them again.

Another reason might be our own fears and uncertainties regarding death. We may never have experienced the death of another or had a near-death experience ourselves, and we do not know what to expect. We are cautious with the person we love because we do not wish to send them into the unknown where we cannot protect and watch over them.

If we are true believers in the Word of God spoken through

the Sacred Scriptures and Sacred Tradition, we should have no fear of the unknown. Every Sunday after the homily we reaffirm those tenets of faith in the Nicene Creed: "I believe in the communion of saints, the forgiveness of sins, the resurrection of the body, and life everlasting." Do you really believe this?

St. Paul tells us, "If our hope in Christ is for this life only, we are the most pitiable people of all."[2] If we as Christians truly believe in the communion of saints and life everlasting with our resurrected bodies, we know that we will see our loved ones again, and should have no hesitation in giving them permission to go home.

Working Out Your Feelings

If you are unsure about letting go, consider the following.

- Pray often and ask God for the wisdom to help you to see clearly in this situation. Pray the Serenity Prayer if you find it helpful to you.
- Talk to your loved one. Ask them if they are ready to go.
- Confront your own fears and hesitations. What is it that is keeping you from letting go? Put a label on it and address the issues one at a time.
- If need be, talk to a pastor, priest, or deacon to help strengthen your belief system about life after death.
- Talk to other siblings and/or members of your family to get their views on the situation.
- Make use of your support systems as recommended in Chapter 2 on the grieving/loss process.
- Trust in the Lord!

An End That Is Just a Beginning

Let go and rejoice, for you will see your loved one again if you live a life rich in Jesus Christ. And at that time, in the new Jerusalem, there will be no more pain, sorrow, or suffering. We are told in the book of Revelation, "He (God) will wipe every tear from their eyes and death shall be no more — no more grief or crying or pain, for what was before has passed away."[3]

Notes

[1] Callanan and Kelley, *Final Gifts*, p. 16.
[2] 1 Cor 15:19.
[3] Rv 21:4.

9

BRINGING IT ALL TOGETHER

"Jesus stopped and called them over and said,
'What do you want me to do for you?' They answered him,
'Lord, let our eyes be opened.'"
(Mt 20:32-33)

It is difficult to deal with the death of a loved one. When that burden is complicated by the decisions you must make on behalf of that loved one, it can become unmanageable, especially if you have 'no clue' as to where to go for the answers. The following issues have been discussed in this guidebook.

SUFFERING

The meaning of suffering was addressed first in this book. As Christians, we are called to suffer with Jesus in order to be glorified with Him. The question we should be asking ourselves is not "Why does God allow suffering?" but "How can I best make use of the suffering I have in the service of God and my brothers and sisters?"

LOSS AND THE GRIEVING PROCESS

All human beings grieve their losses. Grieving is a natural process that helps us to accept the reality of life, viz., that all things die. The fact that we can grieve over the loss of a loved one indicates that a special bond existed between us.

Grieving as a process is dynamic; it flows and is ever changing. There can be progressive healing and periods of regression to a previous stage of grieving. We all grieve differently and recover at different rates. Grieving, like a fingerprint or a snowflake, is unique, and no two individuals grieve in the same manner. Helpful insights are included in Chapter 2 in dealing with loss and the grieving process.

CARE OF THE DYING

This is the hardest ministry you will ever *love!* We might minister easily to others who are dying, but it becomes more difficult the closer to home it becomes.

In Chapter 3 the discussion centers on how best to care for the dying, to deal with the ever-changing emotions of the dying, including the manipulative behavior of the "emotional vampire," and the care of the caregiver. The personal care of the dying can be the most beautiful and rewarding ministry that you accept, but can at the same time be the most stressful and demanding.

RESENTMENT, FORGIVENESS, AND RECONCILIATION

Many family interactions include deep-rooted issues of resentment. These must be resolved if healing is to occur after the death of a loved one. The failure to do so may create additional problems of self-guilt and a sense of having "unfinished business."

Resentment is the hurt that we carry with us over the actions of another person or persons. It eats away at your heart and prevents the love of God from growing within it. Forgiveness releases the wrongdoer from the hold he or she has over you, while not negating or condoning the hurt that has taken place. Forgiveness is one-sided and many times the wrongdoer is not even aware that you have forgiven him or her. We as Christians are required to forgive. If we cannot forgive others' wrongs, how can we accept God's forgiveness of our failings?

Forgiveness that involves both parties is known as reconciliation. Jesus tells us that before we bring our gifts to the altar and remember that we have something against our brother, we are to go first and reconcile with him. This is easy to say but much more difficult to accomplish. When we are able to do so, however, we find that it is the most healing. Reconciliation requires mutual forgiveness and the mutual acceptance of the forgiveness. This type of forgiveness may not always be possible because the person who has hurt us may no longer be present or may even be deceased.

BIO-ETHICAL DECISIONS AND THE TEACHING OF THE CHURCH

If you are a caregiver with durable power of attorney or are responsible for the medical decisions of another, these are probably the most difficult issues to deal with. When is it prudent to start life support and when is it advisable to withdraw it? How can we be sure that we are withdrawing excessively burdensome means of care and not committing euthanasia or assisting in suicide? What does the Church teach us about these matters?

As discussed in Chapter 5, many of these issues are not black and white, but actually very gray in color. They can be difficult decisions to make under the best of conditions, but become horrific nightmares when one is faced with the imminent death of a loved one. Informed ethical decisions *can* be made logically within the teaching guidelines of the Church. It is best to make these decisions with the help of a medical professional and a member of the clergy or a religious.

THE LAST THINGS

The last things are death, judgment, purgatory, hell, and heaven. It is the duty of the caregivers of the dying to help spiritually prepare the loved one for death when they are unable to help themselves to do so.

Death is inevitable and we start dying as soon as we are born. Our lives on earth prepare us for the eternal life following our death. It is important that the dying loved one be able to receive grace through the sacraments. This includes frequent reception of the sacrament of Reconciliation and of the Holy Eucharist. The Church helps us to prepare for death through the administration of the Anointing of the Sick and viaticum. As caregiver, ensure that your loved ones receive these special gifts of grace in preparation for eternal life.

PRAYER

No matter how you feel, prayer is not useless after the diagnosis of a terminal illness. In fact it is quite the contrary. Prayer helps both the caregivers and the dying to prepare for death by coming closer to God. Prayer gives strength, peace, and consolation and helps us to bear life's problems. It is not impossible that a miracle can occur through intercessory prayer; that is why they are called miracles. Miracles occur because people who care pray for them. Prayer is not useless. Pray to God unceasingly. Prayer *is* answered!

SAYING GOODBYE; LETTING GO

When your loved one is ready to die, they will most likely know it. It is important for many dying individuals to be reassured that the family will be able to get along without them and will want to know that it is okay to die. Chapter 8 discusses why a loved one may need permission to "go home" and how a caregiver can give it. It also addresses the issues that may impede a caregiver from saying goodbye and letting go, and some methods to overcome them.

EPILOGUE

It is my hope that, through the grace and inspiration of the Holy Spirit, those who find themselves facing the care of a dying loved one will be helped through this little book. Using my critical care experiences as a nurse, my ministry as a pastoral caregiver, and as one who has had to deal with the painful loss of my own mother to lung cancer, I hopefully have provided some answers to help you during your time of trial and tribulation.

Trust in the Lord and gain your strength from Him through prayer and the sacraments. May God bless you and keep you under the protective mantle of Mary, His holy mother.

BIBLIOGRAPHY

Callanan, M. and P. Kelley, *Final Gifts* (New York: Bantam Books, 1997).

Care of the Sick and Dying (Maryland Catholic Conference of Bishops, Task Force on Medical Decisions, October, 1993).

Carty, C. and L. Rumble, *Why Squander Illness: Prayers and Thoughts for Catholic and Non-Catholic Patients* (Rockford, IL: Tan Books and Publishers, Inc., 1974), p. 33.

Catechism of the Catholic Church (Liguori, MO: Liguori Publications, 1994).

Catherine of Genoa, St., *Fire of Love, Understanding Purgatory* (Manchester, NH: Sophia Institute Press, 1996).

Cloud, H. and J. Townsend, *Boundaries: When to Say Yes and When to Say No To Take Control of Your Life* (Grand Rapids, MI: Zondervan Publishing House, 1992).

Deluxe Bible: The New American Bible. CD-Rom Version 2.0 (Fort Collins, CO: Rocky Mountain Laboratories, 1996).

Frankl, Viktor E., *Meaning of Human Suffering* (Boston: Beacon Press, 1985).

Handbook for Today's Catholic (Liguori, MO: Liguori Publications, 1994).

Hughes, John J., *Centering Prayer: How to Pray From the Heart* (Liguori, MO: Liguori Publishing, 1981).

John Paul II, Encyclical Letter: *Evangelium Vitae,* The Gospel of Life (March 25, 1995).

John Paul II, Apostolic Letter: *Salvifici Doloris*, Salvific Suffering (February 11, 1984).

Lane, Edmund C., SSP, *Do Not Be Afraid, I Am With You,* a book of prayers for those who are shut-in or facing the unknown (New York: Alba House, 1991).

Missinne, Leo E., *How To Find Meaning in Suffering* (Liguori, MO: Liguori Press, 1990).

Moral Issues Regarding Advance Healthcare Directives and Living Wills, Commission for Catholic Life Issues (Los Angeles, CA/Princeton: Scepter Booklets, 1992).

New Testament: St. Paul Catholic Edition (New York: Alba House, 2000).

Niklas, Rev. Gerald R. and Charlotte R. Stefanics, RN, *Ministry to the Sick* (New York: Alba House, 1982).

Niklas, Rev. Gerald R., *The Making of a Pastoral Person* (New York: Alba House, 1996).

O'Donnell, Thomas J., SJ, *Medicine and Christian Morality* (New York: Alba House, 1997).

Pangrazzi, Rev. Arnaldo, *Your Words in Prayer in Time of Illness* (New York: Alba House, 1982).

Pennington, M. Basil, OCSO, *Centering Prayer: Renewing an Ancient Christian Prayer Form* (New York: Image Publishing, 1982).

Schmidt, J., *Praying Our Experiences* (Winona, MN: St. Mary's Press, 1989).

Second Vatican Council, The Constitution on the Sacred Liturgy: *Sacrosanctum Concilium,* December 4, 1963.

Tobin, Eamon, *How to Forgive Yourself and Others* (Liguori, MO: Liguori Press, 1993).

Torok, Lou, *When You Hurt* (New York: Alba House, 1999).

Walsh, James, ed., *The Cloud of Unknowing* (Mahwah, NJ: Paulist Press, 1981).

Wolfelt, Alan D., "Twelve Freedoms of Healing in Grief," *Bereavement Magazine* (February, 1993).

APPENDIX A

Community Resources

HOTLINES

- ALZHEIMER'S ASSOCIATION: (800) 272-3900
- AMERICAN ASSOCIATION OF RETIRED PERSONS (AARP) Information on healthcare treatment and insurance benefits: (800) 424-3410, www.aarp.org
- AMERICAN CANCER SOCIETY: (800) 227-2345, www.cancer.org
- AMERICAN HEART ASSOCIATION Customer Heart And Stroke Information: (800) 242-8721, (800) AHA-USA1
- AMERICAN LUNG ASSOCIATION: (800) 586-4872, (800) LUNG-USA
- AMERICANS WITH DISABILITIES ACT Information and Assistance Hotline: (800) 949-4232
- CANCER HOTLINE: (800) 422-6237, (800) 4-CANCER
- CENTERING CORPORATION, A non-profit bereavement resource center: (402) 553-1200
- CENTERS FOR DISEASE CONTROL AND PREVENTION NATIONAL AIDS HOTLINE: (800) 342-AIDS
- HIV/AIDS TREATMENT INFORMATION SERVICE: (800) 448-0440, tdd: (800) 243-7012
- HOSPICE LINK: (800) 331-1620
- HOSPICE FOUNDATION OF AMERICA: (800) 854-3402 www.hospicefoundation.org
- MEDICARE HOTLINE: (800) 638-6833
- NATIONAL ASSOCIATION FOR HOME CARE [NAHC]: (202) 547-7424 www.nahc.org
- NATIONAL HOSPICE ORGANIZATION [NHO]: (800) 658-8898 www.nho.org
- VISITING NURSE ASSOCIATIONS OF AMERICA [VNA]: (800) 426-2547 www.vnaa.org

SPECIFIC ORGANIZATIONS BY ILLNESS

AIDS/HIV
American Foundation for AIDS Research (AmFAR)
120 Wall Street, 13th Floor
New York, NY 10005
(212) 806-1600

National Association of People with AIDS
1413 K Street NW
Washington, DC 20005
(202) 898-0414

Pediatric AIDS Foundation
2950 31st Street, Suite 125
Santa Monica, CA 90405
(310) 314-1459

ALZHEIMER'S
Alzheimer's Association
National Headquarters
919 N. Michigan Avenue, Suite 1000
Chicago, IL 60611-1676
(800) 272-3900; (312) 335-8700

CANCER
American Cancer Society
1559 Clifton Road NE
Atlanta, GA 30329
(404) 320-3333

Candlelighters Childhood Cancer Foundation
1312 18th Street NW, Suite 200
Washington, DC 20006
(800) 366-CCCF or (202) 659-5136

Make Today Count
101 ½ S. Union Street
Alexandria, VA 22314
(703) 548-9674

CARDIAC/HEART
American Heart Association
National Center
7272 Greenville Avenue
Dallas, TX 75231
Heart and Stroke Information: (800) AHA-USA1

GRIEF MANAGEMENT
GriefNet (Internet community consisting of over 30 e-mail support groups and two websites)
Rivendell Resources
P.O. Box 3272
Ann Arbor, MI 48106-3272
www.Rivendell.org

HOSPICE
Children's Hospice International
1101 King Street, Suite 131
Alexandria, VA 22314
(703) 684-0330

Hospice Net (24-hour Internet service-hospice locator)
401 Bowling Avenue
Nashville, TN 37205-5124
www.hospicenet.org

National Hospice Organization
1901 N. Moore Street, Suite 901
Arlington, VA 22209
(703) 243-5900

LUNGS/PULMONARY
American Lung Association
(800) LUNG-USA
(800) 586-4872

APPENDIX B
Prayers

"Is anyone among you suffering? He should pray."
(Jm 5:13)

Prayers for Guidance

Come, Holy Spirit

Come, Holy Spirit and fill the hearts of your faithful and enkindle in them the fire of your divine love. Send forth your spirit, and they shall be created, and you will renew the face of the earth.

O God, you have instructed the hearts of the faithful by the light of the Holy Spirit. Grant that through the same Holy Spirit we may ever truly be wise and rejoice in his consolation, through Christ Our Lord. Amen.

Prayers for Serenity

Serenity Prayer

God, grant me the serenity to accept the things I cannot change, the courage to change the things I can, and the wisdom to know the difference.

Living one day at a time, enjoying one moment at a time. Accepting hardships as the pathway to peace. Taking as He did, this sinful world as it is, not as I would have it. Trusting that He will make all things right if I surrender to His will; that I may be

reasonably happy in this life and supremely happy with Him forever. Amen. *(Alcoholics Anonymous 12-Step Serenity Prayer)*

Psalm 23

> The Lord is my shepherd;
>   I shall not want.
> In verdant pastures he gives me repose;
>   Beside restful waters he leads me;
> he refreshes my soul.
>   He guides me in right paths
> for his name's sake.
>
> Even when I walk in the dark valley
>   I fear no evil; for you are at my side
> with your rod and your staff
>   that give me courage.
>
> You spread a table before me
>   in the sight of my foes;
> You anoint my head with oil;
>   my cup overflows.
> Only goodness and love follow me
>   all the days of my life;
> And I shall dwell in the house of the Lord
>   for years to come. Amen.

Prayers for Hope

For the Sick

Father, your Son accepted our sufferings to teach us the
virtue of patience in human illness. Hear the prayers we offer for
our sick brother/sister. May all who suffer pain, illness or disease realize that they are chosen to be saints, and know that they
are joined to Christ in His suffering for the salvation of the world,

who lives and reigns with you and the Holy Spirit, one God, forever and ever. Amen.

The Jesus Prayer

Lord Jesus Christ, Son of the living God, have mercy on me, a sinner.

Act of Hope

O my God, relying on your infinite goodness and promises, I hope to obtain pardon of my sins, the help of your grace, and life everlasting, through the merits of Jesus Christ, my Lord and Redeemer. Amen.

Prayer of Hope

My Lord God, I have no idea where I am going. I do not see the road ahead of me. I cannot know for certain where it will end. Nor do I really know myself, and the fact that I think I am following your will does not mean that I am actually doing so.

But I believe that the desire to please you does in fact please you. And I hope I have that desire in all that I am doing. I hope that I will never do anything apart from that desire. And I know that if I do this you will lead me by the right road though I may know nothing about it.

Therefore will I trust you always. Though I may seem to be lost and in the shadow of death, I will not fear, for you are ever with me, and you will never leave me to face my perils alone. Amen. (Thomas Merton, *Thoughts in Solitude*)

Prayer for a Happy Death

My Lord, Jesus Christ, by the bitterness that you endured on the cross when your blessed soul was separated from your most sacred body, have pity on my sinful soul when it leaves my body to enter into eternity.

And you, Mary my Mother, by that grief which you experienced on Calvary in seeing your son Jesus expire on the cross before your very eyes, obtain for me a good death that, through my love in this life for your son Jesus and for you my Mother, I may get to heaven where I shall love you for all eternity. Amen. (St. Alphonsus Liguori)

Prayers for Comfort

Psalm 142
> (A Prayer in Time of Trouble)

With a loud voice I cry out to the Lord;
> with a loud voice I beseech the Lord.
My complaint I pour out before him;
> before him I lay bare my distress.
When my spirit is faint within me,
> you know my path.
In the way along which I walk
> they have hid a trap for me.
I look to the right to see,
> but there is no one who pays me heed.
I have lost all means of escape;
> there is no one who cares for my life.
I cry out to you, O Lord;
> I say, "You are my refuge,
> my portion in the land of the living.
Attend to my cry,
> for I am brought low indeed.
Rescue me from my persecutors,
> for they are too strong for me.
Lead me forth from prison,
> that I may give thanks to your name.

The just shall gather around me
    when you have been good to me."

Prayers for the Departed

Prayer for the Faithful Departed

Eternal rest grant unto them, O Lord, and let perpetual light shine upon them. May their souls and all the souls of the faithful departed, through the mercy of God, rest in peace. Amen.
(An indulgence for the souls in purgatory)

The Rosary

The Joyful Mysteries
- ♦ The Annunciation of Christ's birth to Mary
- ♦ Mary's Visitation to her cousin Elizabeth
- ♦ The Birth of Our Savior
- ♦ The Presentation of the Child Jesus in the Temple
- ♦ The Finding of the Child Jesus in the Temple

The Sorrowful Mysteries
- ♦ Christ's Agony in the Garden
- ♦ His Scourging at the Pillar
- ♦ The Crowning With Thorns
- ♦ Jesus Carries His Cross
- ♦ Jesus Dies on the Cross

The Glorious Mysteries
- ♦ Christ's Resurrection from the dead
- ♦ His Ascension into heaven
- ♦ The Descent of the Holy Spirit on the Apostles
- ♦ The Assumption of Our Lady into heaven
- ♦ The Coronation of Our Lady as Queen of Heaven and Earth

APPENDIX C

How to Pray the "Centering Prayer"

"But when you pray, go to your inner room, close the door, and pray to your Father in secret. And your Father who sees in secret will repay you." (Mt 6:6)

How to Pray the "Centering Prayer"

♦ Pick two times a day when you can devote 15-20 minutes to silent prayer. Upon awakening and before retiring are suggested. Discipline yourself to do this every day, twice a day whether you are in the mood or not. It gets easier and you will see the progress it brings.

♦ Go to a place where you will not be disturbed. A darkened room with a lit votive/prayer candle can set the mood.

♦ Posture is important. Find a comfortable high back chair. You should be comfortable and relaxed sitting upright with your spine straight and your chin off your chest. Breathe deeply, slowly inhaling then exhaling, feeling the rise and the fall of your chest.

♦ Start your prayer with the following antiphon: "O God, come to my assistance; O Lord, make haste to help me." Follow with a favorite Bible verse or Psalm. You may like to recite the prayer "Come Holy Spirit" after the Bible verse.

♦ Close your eyes and clear your mind of any extraneous thoughts. This will be hard to do at times, but it will get easier. To help you to do this, pick a one or two syllable centering word, such as "Jesus" or "Yahweh" or "Lord." When an extraneous thought comes to your mind let it go and quietly repeat the centering word until it disappears. If more thoughts appear, repeat the centering word until they go away.

Think of your mind as a quiet bank next to a moving stream. Things will float downstream to distract you. You look at them, recognize them as a distraction, say the centering word, and let them continue to go downstream away from your view. As other objects come downstream, do the same to them, even if it means you have to do that for the whole twenty minutes. It will get easier and you won't have to repeat the centering word as often.

♦ Do not attempt to pray or engage in two-way conversation with God. Your function is just to sit and listen as the beloved disciple did at the Last Supper to the words of Jesus as He speaks to your heart. If you find that it is almost impossible to focus on keeping quiet, repeat the centering word over and over. Remember that this is the purposeful quiet time that you have set aside to be with Jesus and He appreciates that fact. Even if you become so relaxed that you fall asleep, He still can speak to your heart.

♦ When twenty minutes have elapsed, and this you will know by practicing this prayer many times, slowly say the *Our Father* concentrating on each word and phrase. Then gradually open your eyes. You may wish to conclude with the *Serenity Prayer*.

♦ Until you become accustomed to what twenty minutes of quiet time is, set an alarm in another room just loud enough to let you know when the twenty minutes are up.

♦ You might at first feel this time is useless or wasted, not doing anything at all but listening. But as you will see, insights will come to you as you seek answers from God or his assistance in making decisions. You will wonder where they came from. They came from your heart inspired by Jesus.

This is a cursory introduction to centering prayer. I suggest you get one of many books that address centering prayer and how to pray from the heart. Two such books are:

Centering Prayer: Renewing an Ancient Christian Prayer Form, M. Basil Pennington, OCSO (New York: Image Books, Doubleday & Company, 1980).

Centering Prayer: How to Pray from the Heart, John Jay Hughes, (Liguori, MO: Liguori Publishing, 1981).

A helpful spiritual classic is:

The Cloud of Unknowing, J. Walsh, ed. (Mahwah, NJ: Paulist Press, 1981).

ST PAULS

This book was designed and published by St. Pauls/
Alba House, the publishing arm of the Society of St.
Paul, an international religious congregation of priests
and brothers dedicated to serving the Church through
the communications media. For information regarding
this and associated ministries of the Pauline Family of
Congregations, write to the Vocation Director, Society
of St. Paul, 7050 Pinehurst, Dearborn, Michigan 48126.
Phone (313) 582-3798 or check our internet site,
www.albahouse.org